HEALTH CARE IN TRANSITION

COMPUTING PARADIGMS FOR SMART HEALTHCARE

Health Care in Transition

Additional books and e-books in this series can be found on Nova's website under the Series tab.

HEALTH CARE IN TRANSITION

COMPUTING PARADIGMS FOR SMART HEALTHCARE

B. VINOTH KUMAR
J. UMA MAHESWARI
G. R. KARPAGAM
AND
P. SIVAKUMAR
EDITORS

nova
Medicine & Health
New York

NOTICE TO THE READER

Library of Congress Cataloging-in-Publication Data

ISBN: 978-1-53618-619-2

Published by Nova Science Publishers, Inc. † New York

CONTENTS

PREFACE

Smart healthcare has gradually gained its popularity because of the development of information technologies and computing paradigms such as internet of things (loT), big data, Cloud computing and artificial intelligence. These technologies transform the conventional medical system in to smarter one by making healthcare more convenient, efficient, accurate, and more customized. Smart healthcare will lead to a revolutionized healthcare system that enables the participation of all people for the early prediction and prevention of diseases so that preemptive and pro-active treatment can be delivered.

The aim of this edited book is to publish the latest research advancements in the convergence of automation technology, artificial intelligence, biomedical engineering and health informatics. This will help the readers to grasp the extensive point of view and the essence of the recent advances in this field. This book solicits contributions which include theory, case studies and computing paradigms pertaining to the healthcare applications. The prospective audience would be researchers, professionals, practitioners, and students from academia and industry who work in this field. We hope the chapters presented will inspire future research both from theoretical and practical viewpoints to spur further advances in the field.

The entire book is the contribution of interdisciplinary expertise available in the esteemed Institution PSG College of Technology, an ISO 9001:2015 certified Government aided Institution, belonging to Department of Information Technology, Computer Science and Engineering, Electronics and Communication Engineering, Biomedical Engineering and Biotechnology. A brief introduction about each chapter is as follows.

Chapter 1 focuses on health informatics which provides an overview of the various types of data originating from the medical information,

Chapter 2 objective is to provide a 'smart connected environment' which includes storing, processing and exchange information seamlessly using technologies.

Chapter 3 deals with an intelligent healthcare system for automatic diagnosis of diseases based on IOT enabled cloud computing framework and deep learning

Chapter 4 discuss about basic concepts of digital twin technology and implementation of digital twin in various health care domains.

Chapter 5 proposes a graph based framework for classification, feature selection method which uses the existing notion, histograms for extracting isotonic features from a data set.

Chapter 6 explains the significance of convolution neural network in medical image analysis.

Chapter 7 summarizes recent advances in AI tools applied in cancer diagnosis and research for disease prediction and biomarker discovery.

Chapter 8 explores DNA microarray data followed by the implementation of machine learning algorithms to obtain the highly predictive genes for classification.

Chapter 9 uses various data structures such as hash tables and prefix-based search trees to efficiently query the EHR data present in the Blockchain.

Chapter 10 focuses on agreeing upon a common symmetric cryptographic key generated from the ECG signal collected at different locations of a patient using linear prediction and error control coding techniques.

We are grateful to the authors and reviewers for their excellent contributions for making this book possible.

Dr B Vinoth Kumar
Dr J Uma Maheswari
Dr G R Karpagam
Dr P Sivakumar

July, 2020

In: Computing Paradigms for Smart Healthcare ISBN: 978-1-53618-619-2
Editors: B. Vinoth Kumar et al.

Chapter 1

HEALTHCARE INFORMATICS

R. Vidhyapriya*, PhD and B. Banu Rekha, PhD
Department of Biomedical Engineering,
PSG College of Technology, Coimbatore, India

ABSTRACT

The health care industry is focusing upon value-based business and not on volume-based business, which requires doctors and nurses to be more productive and efficient. Health informaticsalso called as health care information system utilizes the concepts of information engineering to acquire, categorize, manipulate, store and retrieve the health records in order to improve the outcomes / reform healthcare. Health informatics associates information technology, communications and healthcare to improve the quality and safety of patient care. It provides electronic access to medical records of patients.The use of Electronic Health Records (EHR) provides abundant opportunities for data analytics. The structure of EHR, charting the necessary information from EHR will be analyzed in detail. This chapter focuses on health informatics which provides an overview of the various types of data originating from the medical information, an insight into the structure and charting of electronic health records. The analysis of medical data can be utilized in

*Corresponding Author's Email: rvidhyapriya@gmail.com.

providing efficient healthcare through identifying the proper treatment plan and aid in the diagnosis.

Keywords: electronic health record, data analytics, data visualization, healthcare data, data entry points, automated data entry

INTRODUCTION

Healthcare has always been transitional in nature by adapting to emerging technologies and state-of-the art research outcomes. Nevertheless, challenges such as affordability, diseases of unknown etiology and those borne by climatic conditions require large scale collection and analysis of healthcare data. According to the American Medical Informatics Association (AMIA), "Biomedical and health informatics applies principles of computer and information science to the advancement of life sciences research, health professions education, public health, and patient care" [1].

For decades together, genesis of healthcare information took place through oral and handwritten notes. From Papyrus to Electronic Health Records, science and technology has revolutionized the way healthcare information is recorded, transmitted and analyzed. The focus of healthcare has shifted from curing diseases to providing point-of-care solutions that is attributed to the convergence of digital technologies and advanced communication systems. Decision support sytems and data mining methods are built on humongous amount of data rendered by e-health systems and wearable's. The global digital healthcare industry is estimated to reach$224 billion by 2023[2].

The organization of this chapter is as follows. The first section of this chapter presents an overview of the healthcare data and the variety ofsources from which the data is generated. The section also provides a comprehensive coverage of the types of medical data and the various points of its entry into a typical Information system. The second section on Electronic Health Record (EHR) gives an overview of the data-driven appraoch that integrates EHR with Clinical Informatics Systems and the Nursing Informatics Systems. The third section provides the methods and tools used in analysis and visualization of healthcare data. The concluding section presents the data analytics approaches such as exploratory, descriptive, diagnstic, predictive and prescriptive with real life examples.

OVERVIEW OF HEALTHCARE DATA

Data are obtained through observations and they are typically unprocessed. The observations could be manual, viz. a physician looking for certain symptoms or signs to evaluate the health condition of a subject. Observations could arise from a medical equipment, such as a CT or MRI image of a patient. Observations could also stem from an instrument viz. administering a questionnaire about the underlying health conditions of a patient under consultation. Finally, observations can also be collected from automated systems such as wearable's designed to measure and transmit signals dynamically.

Data that is analyzed and interpreted using scientific and mathematical methods is considered as information. Knowledge is gained when information about the past and present conditions along with the current data are built together.Knowledge is essential in a decision making process. Figure 1 depicts these relationship visually. Artificial Intelligence based decision assist devices and algorithms are needed in nearly all the aspects of diagnosis and treatment.

Healthcare Data Resources

Healthcare and medical care are used synonymously in healthcare literature. While medical data is about the diagnosis, treatment and prognosis and other services offered by healthcare providers,healthcare data is a larger term encompassing the medical data along with administrative data and business oriented healthcare data. Healthcare data are acquired from the following seven resources [3].

- Surveys
- Administrative and medical records
- Claims data
- Vital records
- Surveillance
- Disease registries
- Peer-reviewed literature

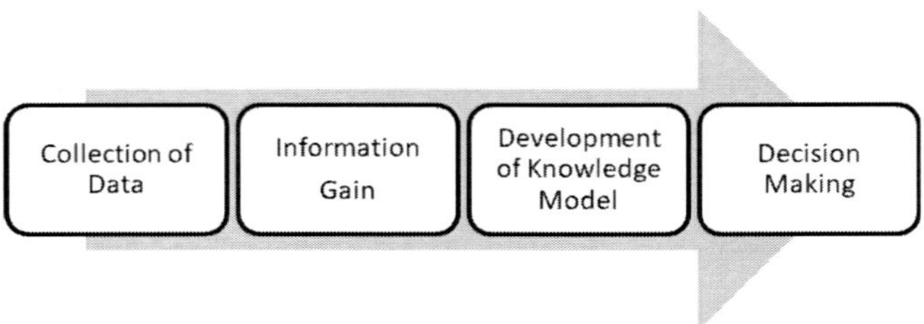

Figure 1. Stages involved in Clinical Decision Assist Methods.

Surveys

Surveys are used to collect information about a sample of people among a larger population. The surveys can be in the form of questionnaires, personal interaction, telephonic and email interviews. While the success of surveys depends on many factors such as how much it is unbiased, how quickly it is conceived after a particular event, and its validity, the primary factor is the proper designing of the survey.

Administrative and Medical Records

Medical records are used to improve the quality of healthcare and support patient care. Electronic records have the advantage of delivering legible information, quick updating of data and ability to create charts and trends for caregivers. The components of a medical record are the medical history, present findings, test results and information related to the treatment procedure. Medical record formats are classified into two types:

- Source-Oriented Medical Record (SOMR)
- Problem-Oriented Medical Record (POMR)

SOMR is a traditional and chronological medical record. It has specific sections for data entry and generally cross referencing of data across sections are not possible [4]. POMR is a modernized version of medical record. While SOMR is designed based on the needs of personnel entering data, POMRprovides better structure and organization to assist those reading and using the data. Electronic Health Records are dealt in detail in the subsequent chapter.

Administrative records contain information such as demographics, insurance details, legal information and correspondence. These records are generally arranged in a reverse chronological manner. While administrative records are primarily used for management purposes, they play a major role in insurance billing, assessment of healthcare and public health policy making. An emerging discipline of healthcare information management system concerns with the acquisition, evaluation and up keeping of medical records in accordance with policies and standards such as HIPAA, IHE, HL7.

Claims Data

Medical Claims include diagnosis codes, procedural codes, site of service details, specialty of the providers and other revenue related items. From the healthcare payer's perspective, claims data is the primary information about billing and services including pharmacy claims [5]. These data are made available at all healthcare sites such as inpatient and outpatient hospitals, Emergency Rooms, surgical and laboratory centers and the physician's office.

Vital Records

Vital records provide government with details of life events such as birth, death and marital status. Ill fated incidents such as foetal death and still births are also recorded. These records help in assessing the effectiveness of healthcare measures undertaken by governments.

Mortality statistics is significant to improve the public health of a country Vital records also serve a larger purpose in understanding the socio economic implications of maternity and child care.

Surveillance

Healthcare surveillance is the close observation and monitoring of healthcare information, mostly used in the context of public health informatics. The data is analyzed and disseminated at appropriate time to prevent and control diseases. Databases are maintained at designated offices and are periodically updated through electronic reporting systems.

Surveillance technologies get impetus during outbreaks, notably, the recent COVID-19, declared as pandemic by the WHO. A situation dashboard was designed by WHO as shown in Figure 2. Data from various countries were added to the database on a per day basis. The dashboard was a source of evidence based data and it provided users with the options of creating charts and trend lines according to region, country or continent.

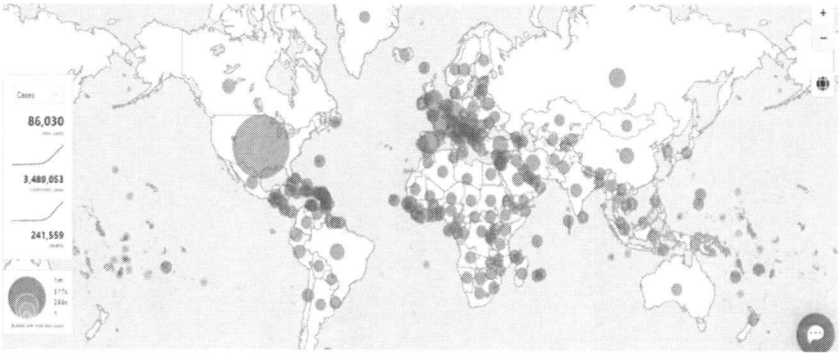

Figure 2. COVID-19 situation Dashboard, designed by WHO.

Drones poised to be disruptors for healthcare surveillance. They are essential in the times of chemical and biological hazards [6]. They were designed to be disinfectant sprayers, medical supply delivery and carry out surveillance to ensure social distancing.

Disease Registries

Disease registry is a special type of database that contains information about a specific disease among a large population. The purpose of creating and maintaining disease registry is either scientific, clinical or policy making. The registry can be hospital based or population based. A hospital based registry maintains data about a specific disease treated within the hospital. A population registry maintains data about people diagnosed with a specific disease within a geographical area. These registries support patient care activities such as treatment and follow up, continuing education for self management and personalized care.

Some of the prominent registries in India are The National Cancer Registry Programme, The National Injury Surveillance & Trauma Registry, Neonatal and Maturity onset of youth registry, Clinical Trials Registry India andNational Stroke Registry Programme.

Peer-Reviewed Literature

Peer-reviewed literature presents results of evidence based research that are systematically conducted following the scientific guidelines. Peer review done by expert scholars make sure that the quality of research is high and contributes to the scientific community. In a study conducted to identify the high impact health informatics literature [7], the following categories wereapplied to classify literature: EHRs, clinical Decision Support Systems (CDSS), computerized provider order entry (CPOE), electronic prescribing (eRx), health information exchange (HIE), patient safety, standards and interoperability, adoption strategies, business case, evaluation studies in health IT and workflow analysis.

Types of Medical Data

Medical data consists of observations and measurements recorded during regular patient care. From the perspective of data analytics, it is important to classify medical data such that appropriate algorithms can be built to operate on them. The major classifications of medical data are given below. A detailed discussion is provided on each of these categories.

- Numerical data
- Categorical data
- Structured data
- Unstructured data

Numerical Data

Numerical Data are those that can be measured using medical devices. Numerical data can further be classified as continuous and discrete data. While the term 'continuous' can point to a time series data such as a bio signal, the real context of this term is the infinite number of values that may occur within a selected range.

The test results of majority of the pathology tests are continuous in nature. Pathology tests are done on blood, urine, faeces and biopsy samples. Table 1 and Table 2 lists some of the continuous medical data. The ranges indicated are suggestive and are not intended to give clinical advice.

Table 1. Numerical continuous data

Type of Test	Range (Suggestive Examples)
Albumin	35 to 50 g/l
Proteinin Serum	6 to 8 g/dl
Protein in Urine	0 to 14 mg/dL
Bilirubin Level	0.1 to 1.2 mg/dL
Random Blood Glucose	4.4–7.8 mmol/l
Blood pH	7.35 to 7.45
Body Mass Index	18.5 to 25
Hematocrit	38.3-44.9 percent

Discrete numerical data are those having distinct or particular values. Counts such as red blood cell count, platelet count and rates of certain bio signals fall under this category.

Table 2. Numerical discrete data

Type of Test	Range (Suggestive Examples)
White Blood Cell Count	3.4 - 9.6 billion cells/L
Platelet count	135-317 billion/L
Urine Culture	1,000 to 10,000 CFU/mL
Respiratory Rate	12 - 20 breaths per min
Blood Oxygen Level	95 - 100 percent
Resting heart rate	60 - 100 beats per min

Categorical Data

Certain types of medical data have a fixed number of possible values. The data value will take any one of the predetermined categories. These are known as Categorical data. Categorical data are classified as Nominal and Ordinal data. A Nominal data does not have any innate ordering, which means, the categories are unique and distinct but doesn't follow any relation between them. Tables 3 and 4 provide few examples of these type of categorical data.

Table 3. Categorical nominal data

Type of Test	Categories (Suggestive Examples)
Blood Grouping	A, B, AB, O
Gender	M, F, Other
Marital Status	Married, Unmarried, Divorcee
Readmitted Status	Yes, No
Emotional States	Anger, Fear, Disgust, Happy, Sad, Surprise, Neutral
Anomaly Scan	Normal, Abnormal

Table 4. Categorical ordinal data

Type of Test	Categories (Suggestive Examples)
Mitotic Rate in CA test	1,2,3
Tumor Grade	1,2,3,4
Liver Cirrhosis	Mild, Moderate, Severe
Brain Activity	Alpha, Beta, Gamma, Theta, Delta
Parkinson's Disease	Stages 1,2,3,4,5
Diabetic Retinopathy	Mild nonproliferative retinopathy, Moderate nonproliferative retinopathy, Severe nonproliferative retinopathy, Proliferative retinopathy

Structured Data

In the previous sections, data as a separate entity was discussed. The data had properties and were measurable. In a complex field such as healthcare, data are bound together in the form of a record. A single data or a data type cannot be a potential indicator of a health condition. For any specific procedure such as registration, discharge, test, diagnosis or treatment, a cluster of healthcare data are needed. In order to create a detailed record that is suitable for transfer among different healthcare information systems, standard data fields and formats are needed. Such a record is a valuable asset as it can be stored for further analysis.

Electronic Health Records are an excellent source of structured medical data. The data elements include the medical diagnosis, signs and symptoms, tests and procedures, prescription and insurance details. To enable interoperability, it is advised to follow standard nomenclature and codes such as SNOMED - CT and ICD.

Unstructured Data

Unstructured data does not conform to any pre-determined format. It is an information that consists of text, dates, multimedia content and handwritten notes. About 80% of the medical data is in unstructured form [8]. Majority of this data such as signal, images do not reach the structured data records. Latest researches conducted in healthcare field using artificial intelligence techniques and big data perspectives need to mine these form of unstructured data. Hence, measures are required to properly define, extract, standardize and visualize the unstructured data.

Healthcare Databases

A database is an organized collection of structured information, or data, typically stored electronically in a computer system [9]. Since healthcare data is voluminous and consists of various formats such as numerical, categorical, structured and unstructured, database management system (DBMS) becomes essential. R.D. Lele [10] describes four types of databases as applicable to the field of healthcare: Patient databases, Hospital databases, Nationwide databases andKnowledge databases.

Patient databases are a collection of events, encounters, procedure and billing details of a single patient. The purpose of such a database is to provide personalized healthcare, reduce medical errors, enable hassle-free insurance and billing services and for statistical analysis. Hospital databases are maintained by an individual hospital or a chain of hospitals. These are generally taken care by third party providers. It requires an intense infrastructure to properly store sensitive medical information with adequate safety measures. Nationwide databases are built by governmental organizations for the wider purpose of policy making and planning. These databases are chiefly used for driving healthcare strategies during epidemics and pandemics. Knowledge databases are peer reviewed and validated medical literature that researchers and practitioners regard. The concept of evidence based medicine substantially relies on these knowledge databases.

Data Entry Points in a Typical Clinical Setting

Workflow analysis tracks the set of tasks involved in a process and identifies the personnel and resources involved in these tasks.To analyze the data entry points in a healthcare organization, workflow analysis is needed. The analysis can be done at three levels: inter-organizational, within the organization and individual cognitive level. The current discussion revolves around the workflow within a healthcare organization and the entry points for recording the patient data. Hence, a workflow analysis from the perspective of a patient is needed. A typical patient workflow is shown in Figure 3.

Patient workflow in a typical healthcare provider organization begins with the patient reporting to the hospital. After reporting to the front office, they are classified as old, revisited or new patients. A patient record is created for every new patient registered. The insurance details are also for revisiting patients, medical history and follow up instructions are recorded.

For old patients, the current complaints and presenting symptoms are registered.

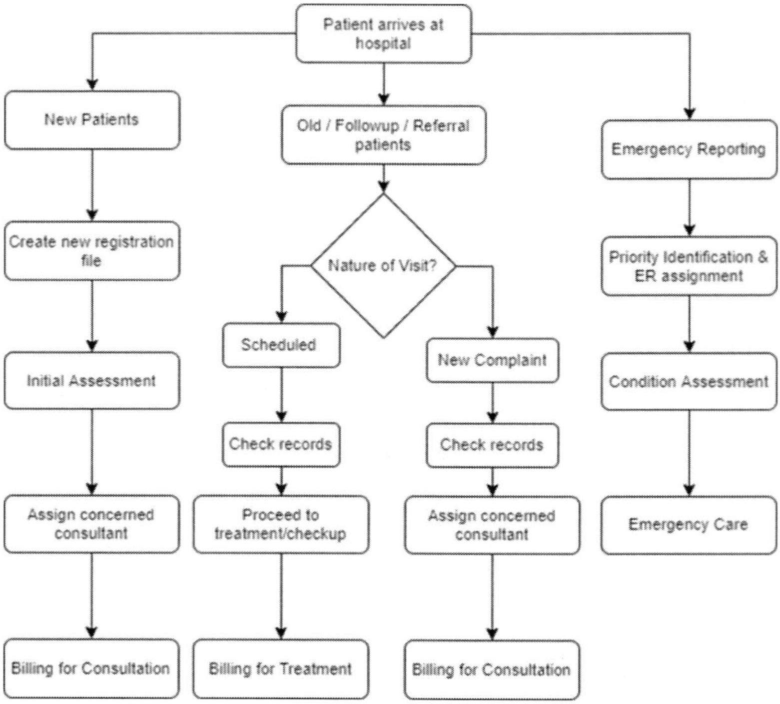

Figure 3. A typical patient workflow.

During consultation, tests are ordered by the physician to confirm diagnosis. The procedures are ordered through Hospital Information System (HIS) and routed through Laboratory Information System (LIS). The test results are enteredinto the record along with the summary of diagnosis and treatment procedure initiated. Based on the lab test results, the procedure may be continued, changed or terminated. These changes are also recorded as data in the patient record.

Apart from laboratory based tests, the physicians would order for imaging and bio signal recording of the patients based on the signs and symptoms. In some situations, more than one type of tests are ordered to confirm the primary diagnosis. The observations and summary of the findings by the physician is another entry point of the data that takes form as unstructured data.

Prescription of drugs is an integral part of a patient record. Prescription of drugs can be done in two ways: prescribing to an inpatient and prescribing to a home based patient. In patients can be advised on drugs through entry into their patient records and connecting it to the HIS. Home based patients can be advised through email communication or through the HIS that has a separate patient portal.

Hospital Information Systems contain a module for insurance and billing. With the implementation of electronic health records, it has become easier to link the medical billing module with the patient details. Billable services are linked to the healthcare delivery procedure to provide a hassle free and transparent billing process.From the billing module, it should be able to generate and approve payments, and analyze payments based on various criteria such as insurance providers, healthcare providers and insurance beneficiaries.

Discharge data is the concluding data of a hospitalization event. Discharge summaries need to adhere to guidelines. These guidelines mention which content of e-data should be entered into the discharge summary. The importance of discharge summary is that it narrates the entire patient care plan. It is critical to care givers post-hospitalization and while getting readmitted to the same healthcare provider or another provider.

Automated Capture and Recording of Medical Data

The simplest and most powerful method for automated recording of data is through creation of questionnaires and forms that are filled by the patients. While emergency rooms cannot expect the patients to fill these forms on their arrival, this method will suit the patients who are not admitted on an urgent basis. The major fields in a self-reported patient admission form are:

- Basic demographic details such as name, age, gender, marital status and ethnicity
- Location and contact details such as postal address, pin code primary and secondary contact details and email id.
- Individual details such as blood type, unique ID (SSN, UIDAI), and occupation
- Insurance details such as provider, plan covered under, relationship, and employer details.

The scope for automation lies in the front office infrastructure. The front office software should have facilities to send pre-intake forms to the patients identified as visitors. Even when they report freshly to the hospital, they would be handed mobile devices to enter the basic data required for front office. These steps are needed to reduce errors in data entry, pre validate insurance, easy and instant integration with the HIS, get the consent of patients in digital form. The vital details collected during the front office encounter has a profound impact on the health outcome. A recent study [11] has found that demographics, preexisting health and acute illness severityact as determinants of health-related quality of lifepost ICU.

Barcode scanners enable faster and accurate method of data entry in hospitals. Patient IDs are critical in a healthcare setting in which a slight change of numbers could result in fatalities. Hence, an efficient way to identify patients is to tag them with a barcode tag and use scanners every time a procedure such as routine checkup, imaging test, laboratory tests are performed. The barcode scanner can automatically upload the patient id to the patient record in order to update the record. Scanners are commonly available in two formats: 1D and 2D. 1D barcode uses patterns of shapes and dots to uniquely identify things while 2D barcodes have alphanumeric data, URLs, images etc. 3D barcodes have also come into existence that has color as an added dimension.

Laboratory Information Systems (LIS) are coupled with HIS to provide access to physicians in ordering tests faster and to get the results back in time to aid diagnosis and treatment. While time to obtain results is crucial, it is equally important to provide validated results. An automatic system for verification, validation and delivery of laboratory results was developed [12] and it achievedreduced manual data entry and increased the timeliness and utility of test results.

ELECTRONIC HEALTH RECORDS

Computerization of health care system began nearly sixty years ago with the invention of computers. Pioneer of healthcare informatics, Dr. Morris F. Collen predicted the huge impact of computers in the field of healthcare. He was instrumental in creating a first-of-its kind multiphasic health record. Electronic Health Record (EHR) is a key milestone that has revolutionized healthcare in the last decade. According to ISO/TS 18308: 2004, thestandard on Health informatics Requirements for an Electronic Health Record Architecture, EHR has similar names such as Electronic Medical Record (EMR), Electronic Patient Record (EPR),Computerized Patient Record or Computer-based Patient Record (CPR),Electronic Health Care Record (EHCR), Virtual EHR, Personal Health Record (PHR) and Digital Medical Record (DMR). Even though functionally similar, there are slight changes between them that depend on the region or manufacturer. As early as 1997, ASTM (American Society for Testing and Materials) has developed and published ASTM E1384-96 Standard Guide for Content and Structure of the Computer-Based Patient Record[13].This standard guide was intended to provide the framework vocabulary for the computer-based patient record content.This standard outlined the many advantages of EHRs [14].

- a unified repository of healthcare information
- information that is accessible from multiple sites
- more efficient communication between healthcare providers
- cross-patient retrievals will provide statistics needed by clinical, outcomes, and health service researchers as well as administrators and managers

- better defined policies and procedures to improve healthcare practice
- a longitudinal health record that can be developed more efficiently and effectively
- The advantages of having standards for the content design in EHRs are mentioned as follows.
- providing a clear description of the data elements that will be included in an EHR
- identifying essential data elements such as temperature and blood pressure
- standardizing the field length, data type, and content of each data field
- improving the degree of granularity
- accommodating varying degrees of granularity in the recording of the same clinical information within one patient's record
- accommodating both structured and free-text reporting
- relating the major entities of the record to the identified record segments
- matching data elements across systems for extensive patient care reporting, overall improvement in the quality of patient care, and the development of a longitudinal health record

The ASTM E1633 Standard was used to specify coded values used in EHRs. The intention of this standard was to create unified representations for the data elements primarily present in EHR and those that are derived from them.It emphasized on exchangeable patient care. It created an avenue to the concept of interoperability that is much debated in the current health scenario.

The ISO 13606 standard was designed by European Committee for Standardization (CEN) in 2008[15]. The objective of the ISO 13606 standard was to define a rigorous and stable information architecture for communicating part or all of the electronic health record (EHR) of a single subject of care (patient) between EHR systems, or between EHR systems and a centralized EHR data repository.

The Government of India notified EHR Standards for India in 2013. It underwent revision and was published again as EHR Standards for India, 2016 [16]. The standards were supported by professional bodies, regulatory bodies, stakeholders and various technical and social commentators. The EHR gets defined as "*An Electronic Health Record (EHR) is a collection of various medical records that get generated during any clinical encounter or events.*" EHR is considered to substantially increase personal and public health.

The current challenges of healthcare data collection are manifold: to provide evidence based care, faster and accurate diagnosis, personalized healthcare through analytics and a platform for improved policy making. While EHRs can generate mountains of data, the need is to create clinically significant and meaningful summary of the events. It is a fact that there is no one-size-fits-all EHR solution. It was noted that various vendors had separately developed EHR systems that formatted data in different ways, which made it hard to share records between hospitals, physicians and external testing laboratories [17]. But, interoperability is the only way ahead to share the records across healthcare establishments. EHRs also come with certain disadvantages. It has been accused of bringing 'burn-outs' in physicians due to longer times spent on EHRs to enter patient data. In turn, the meaningful message conveyed to the physician is sparse while compared to the effort spent on feeding the data. Hence, Artificial Intelligence techniques are now used on EHRs to churn out data in a way that can aid physicians in faster and accurate decision-making. Another engrossing research being conducted using EHR data is the development of Precision medicine. Precision medicine is the targeted delivery of personalized medicine based on the genetic profile of the patients. In the existing EHR systems, certain interpretations from whole genome sequencing are recorded as allergies, such that it can be considered during drug prescription. Knowledge about WGS-derived variants would become essential with pharmacogenomics backed diagnosis and treatment [18].

The rest of this section details the typical structure of an EHR, denoting the front end and back end components. We then discuss about how the EHR data is used to create visualizations and trends. Dashboards are being increasingly designed to show the real time status of patients. Further, chronic illness conditions and communicable disease spread need visualizations for tracking and decision making. Finally, the section ends with a discussion on the recent advances in the Clinical and Nursing Informatics specialties. The success of EHR implementation and interoperability are dependent on these informatics applications.

Structure and Standards of EHR

The structure of EHR is varied according to the specifications of various vendors who develop these applications. Two main semantic standards used in structuring of EHRs are the openEHR and HL7. The two standards are explored in this section.

OPENEHR Based Electronic Health Records

openEHR is the name of a technology for e-health, consisting of open specifications, clinical models and software that can be used to create standards, and build information and interoperability solutions for healthcare[19]. It is a community driven effort to provide an open model. The semantic framework of EHR is represented inFigure 4. A Semantic Framework provides a knowledge based approach to the architecture of EHRs. While we are discussing the framework of an open standard EHR, nevertheless, it represents the backbone of a wider variety of EHR solutions. Reference models have to be adopted for representing the data in EHR. It is essential that adherence to standard terminologies cater to interoperability. A Detailed Clinical Model (DCM) is one such approach in which components such as Clinical knowledge specification, Data element specification and Meta data specification are discretely categorized [20].

Archetype Definition Language (ADL), Unified Modeling Language (UML) and/or eXtensible Markup Language (XML) are the common specification methods assumed by various models.

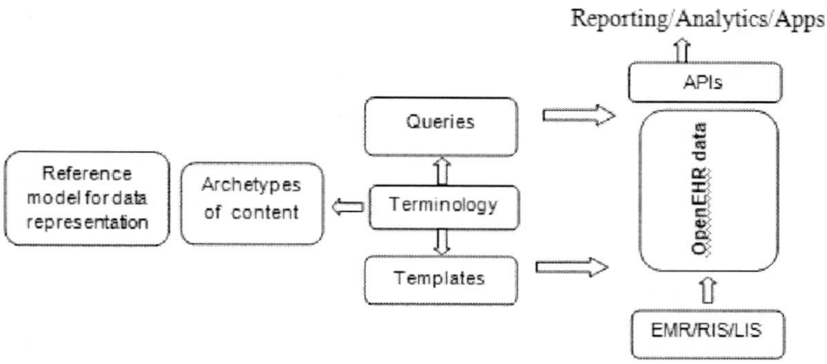

Figure 4. Simplified Semantic Framework of OpenEHR.

The archetypes define the standardized content specification that is handled by the EHR based on the specific topic or a theme. The archetypes are derived from the reference data models. Examples of Archetypes such as Apgar result and Blood pressure measurement actually contain data points relevant to the result measured. Archetypes are assembled using templates. The slots in the templates are filled with archetypes of a particular relationship hierarchy and function as library. The templates help in composition, element choosing, narrowing search constraints and setting default values.

OpenEHR supports two kinds of terminology: external and internal. The internal terminology takes a form of a set of {code, text, description} for each and every node of the archetype structure. Node has a unique id in the structure from which a leaf may occur (branching ontology). External terminology refers to the recognized terminologies such as SNOMED-CT (Systematized Nomenclature of Medicine -- Clinical Terms), LOINC(Logical Observation Identifiers Names and Codes), ICD(International Classification of Diseases), ICPC (International Classification of Primary Care)etc. SNOMED-CT provides clinical concepts and logical definitions as a vocabulary. LOINC is a standard for representing, observations and measurements. ICD and ICPC provide systematically derived codes for medical conditions. These external terminologies are highly sought after for providing interoperability in EHR systems.

A general model of recording healthcare events in openEHR is represented in Figure 5. The health care events are reported as entries based on certain constraints. The clinical statements are recorded at the time of theirhappening, while thehealthcare events are sampled and eventually recorded. While multiple events are recorded using electronic devices and computers, it is insightful to record only the data events at certain data points that enable diagnosis or bring a change in the diagnosis or treatment procedure.

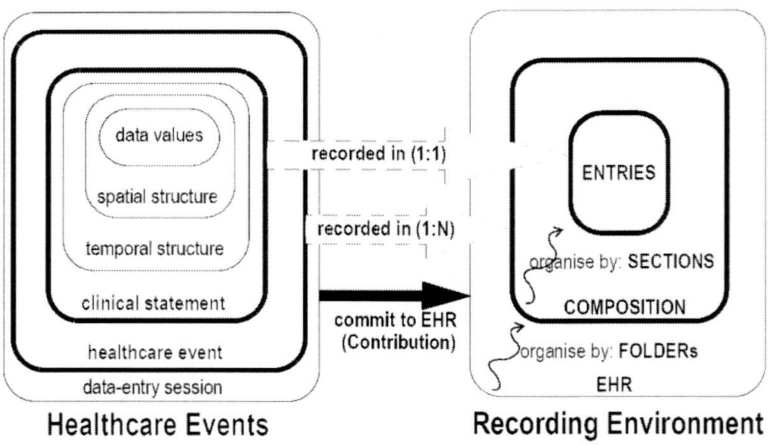

Figure 5. General Model of Recording in openEHR [21].

Query languages such as SQL, OQL and XQuery are popular for database management systems. Yet, they are not compatible with all types of data schemas and data representations. Hence, Archetype Query Language (AQL) is used in openEHR. The queries are made up of a combination of semantic elements and data structure elements. Appropriate APIs are used to convert the data into formats suitable for Apps, reporting structures and programs that perform analytics. The data is collected from Electronic Medical Records, Hospital Information System, Laboratory Information System and Radiology Information System.

HL7 Based Electronic Health Records

Health Level Seven International (HL7) is an technical organization that provides a '*comprehensive framework and related standards for the exchange, integration, sharing, and retrieval of electronic health information that supports clinical practice and the management, delivery and evaluation of health services*' [22].The mission of HL7 standards is to make global health data interoperable. HL7 is a messaging standard and it defines the structure of messages and documents that are shared or exchanged in XML format. HL7 has defined a architecture for clinical documents that is called Clinical Document Architecture (CDA).A Continuity of Care Document (CCD) defines the minimum set of clinical data to be shared or exchanged between healthcare providers.A typical HL7 message appearsas given here.

```
MSH|^~\&|ADT1|MCM|LABADT|MCM|198808181126|SECURITY|
ADT^A01|MSG00001-|P|2.6EVN|A01|198808181123
PID|||PATID1234^5^M11^^AN||JONES^WILLIAM^A^III||19610615|
M||2106-3|677
DELAWARE AVENUE^^EVERETT^MA^02149|GL|(919)379-1212|
(919)271-3434~(919)277-3114||S||PATID12345001^2^M10^^ACSN|
123456789|9-87654^NC
NK1|1|JONES^BARBARA^K|SPO|||||20011105
NK1|1|JONES^MICHAEL^A|FTH
PV1|1|I|2000^2012^01||||004777^LEBAUER^SIDNEY^J.|||SUR||-
||ADM|A0
AL1|1||^PENICILLIN||CODE16~CODE17~CODE18
AL1|2||^CAT DANDER||CODE257
IN1|001|A357|1234|BCMD|||||132987
IN2|ID1551001|123456789
```

The message consists of segment labels that are three-lettered words. In the above example, the segment labels are MSH (Message Header),

EVN (Event Type), PID (Patient Identification), NK1(Next of Kin), PV1(Patient Visit), AL1(Allergy), and IN1 (Insurance).

The HL7 International EHR System Functional Model (EHR-S FM) created a layout for features and functions accommodated in EHR systems. EHR-S FM is not a specification by itself, but it contributes to the development of a longitudinal health record. It has 320 functions along with 2300 conformance criteria. The EHR-S Functional Model consists of a set of Functions and their associated Functional Descriptors. These functions are divided into three sections: Direct Care, Supportive, and Information Infrastructure [23]. The Direct Crae section refers to functions that provide direct healthcare or direct self-care to onee or more persons. The Supportive functions are the group of functions that frequently use data from EHRs. The Information Infrastructure functions are the critical backbone elements of security, privacy, interoperability, registry and vocabulary. The functions are selected and customized for a particular application, setting, user, domain etc. The functions are prioritized as Essential Now, Essential Future, Optional and Not Applicable/Supported.

HL7 Reference Information Model (RIM) has six main classes, Act, Entity, Role, ActRelationship, Participation and RoleLink. Act refers to actions and events that arise out of health care services. Entities represent a group of classes of the stakeholders. Role defines on the functions performed by participants in an event. The other three, ActRelationship, Participation and RoleLink contain classes that focus on the various participation and relation between acts.

FHIR (Fast Healthcare Interoperability Resources)

FHIR (Fast Health Interoperability Resources) is an HL7 specification for Healthcare Interoperability[24]. FHIR is a combination of the best features of existing standards for EHR. EHRs from various vendors store data in different ways locally. FHIR focuses on implementation and is able to provide healthcare quality measures related data. electronic clinical quality measure (eCQM) is the clinical quality measure that uses data from

EHR that are recorded in a structured form. eCQM consists of three parts: Data model, expression logic and structure. FHIR resource is a pair of standard definitions and descriptions on using the resource in a human readable format. Similar to openEHR and HL7, FHIR resources can be customized that are called profiles.

EHR Standards for India

The EHR standards for India (2016 version) provides key standards for the following components of HER [25].

- Identification & Demographics
- Patient Identifiers
- Architecture Requirements
- Functional Requirements
- Reference Model and Composition
- Terminology
- Coding System
- Imaging
- Scanned or Captured Records
- Data Exchange
- Discharge/Treatment Summary
- E-Prescription
- Personal Healthcare and medical Device Interface
- Data Privacy and Security
- Information Security Management
- Privilege Management and Access Control
- Audit Trail and Logs
- Data Integrity
- Data Encryption
- Digital Certificate

While each of these components are governed by the corresponding standards, the true sense of interoperability lies in connecting layers of network transportation, description of data and services, reference information models, vocabularies and codes.

Charting of EHR Data

A chart is a collection of data presented in a graphical form. While most of charts represent numerical data in tabulated form, some forms of charts can also represent qualitative data that are systematically collected. EHRs are also a form of chart that is in electronic form. Within EHRs, charts are used to record the notes rendered by physicians that track the progress. Charts are considered as legal documents. Charts can also be preserved for future studies and research.

EHRs store longitudinal data that spanmultiple years. A simple way to understand the spread of data is to perform visualization. The data pertaining to multiple visits of patients, the changing nature of medical problems, medications, treatments and prognosis are better illustrated through innovative methods by researchers. LifeLines was one of the earliest visualization endeavours [26]. The personal history of juveniles were presented as trends in a streamline fashion. The project enabled spotting of anomalies among the data and locating missing information was a consequence of the analysis. The CNTRO time-relation reasoning framework was designed to semantically represent relations and constraints in EHR data [27]. Clinical Narrative Temporal Relation Ontology that models temporal function from structure data as well as data in natural language formats. It was modeled in Web Ontology Language (OWL) format. A demonstration was done to reveal temporal patterns from a large database of EHRs [28]. The study created interpretable associations. A multivariate clustering approach, Radial Domain Folding (RDF) [29] was used to visualize patient states from data collected through EHRs. In the RDF technique, data from nearly 100 dimensional space was used to capture the severity level with which each organ is affected. The data was also used to predict the mortality of patients who fell at the high severity level.

Patient similarity analytics were used to identify a group of patients who were similar to a target patient. The visual cluster models were used to generate patient cohorts [30]. An interactive visualization tool, DICON, enabled users to manipulate the clusters. Dashboards are an innovative way of representing EHR data. In aresearch work that focused on two areas, namely, sepsis patient outcomes and 30-day hospital readmissions,dashboards were developed with the goal of aggregating data and providing meaningful summary statistics, highlighting critical performance metrics, and providing easily digestible visuals that can be understood by a wide range of personnel with varying levels of skill and areas of expertise [31]. This dashboard improved the efficiency of healthcare, by saving the precious time of providers. Anintegrated visualization of EHR data was designed according to the two dimensional act-time relationships [32]. A comparative study of 8 systems that could graphically display diagnostic test results in electronic health records was performed [33]. It was found that only two EHR systems allowed users to see, hover-over, or click on a data point to see the precise values of the x-y coordinates. The study concluded that user interaction in these type of visualization systems are needed for optimal use of the graphs.

EHR in Clinical Informatics

Clinical informatics deals with the application of informatics and informatics tools in the delivery of healthcare. It combines information science, systems, knowledge management and workflow analysisto support healthcare professionals. Since most of modern clinical data emerges from EHRs, it is imperative that EHRs play an important role in the successful outcome of clinical informatics. While clinical informatics is primarily data-driven, other applications include patient identification & tracking using RFID tags, bed management and creation of electronic portals.

For a health system that learns by itself, an ecosystem has to be created that is integrated, interoperable and robust. For this to happen, EHR data has to be transformed into knowledge. Every event and encounter that is recorded on an EHR can provide an opportunity to gain insights on the healthcare. Based on a study conducted among on the reuse perspectives of EHRs by clinicians among the recent literature, eight types of data content were suggested to be addedto EHRs in the future. These were Adverse Events, Clinician Cognitive Processes, Data Standards Creation and Data Communication, Genomics, Medication List Data Capture, Patient Preferences, Patient-reported Data, and Phenotyping [34]. Thus will enable the need of advanced analytical requirements.

American Medical Informatics Association (AMIA) has created a Task Force on the status and future direction of EHRs [35]. The Task Force addressed five areas and ten recommendations.

- Reduce the burden of data entry for the clinicians
- Data entry and reporting to be executed separately
- Research in the field of healthcare and new learnings about healthcare should be enabled by EHRs is a systematic method through various methods of capturing and reporting the clinical data.
- Focused outcomes through implementation of regulationstandards.
- Innovations and creative changes in EHR systems to be supported through regulations.
- Certified EHR Technology (CEHRT) is used to evaluateEHR applications. These certifications have to be made flexible and transparent.
- Risk assessment and declarations should be made transparent. Risk mitigation strategies to be practiced through collaboration.
- Extend the EHR scope from clinical use to societal health by considering home based healthcare, entities like laboratory, pharmacy, long-term care, community health, private therapy practitioning etc.

- Understand the need for user-interface design based on cognitive needs.

EHR in Nursing Informatics

Nursing Informatics isthe field that integrates nursing science and informatics to provide better healthcare to individual patients, population and communities. Nursing Informaticist is an evolving career that researches, educates and promotes applications of informatics and informatics tools. Nursing jobs require foundational skills such as professionalism, compassion, time management and communication. The skills required to function in an electronic environment is the awareness of technologies, attention to details of the system, critical thinking, identification of grey areas of ICT applications and following the principles of ethics.

A study was conducted on the electronic nursing documentation and its effects on the quality of healthcare[36]. The study included literature on quality of care provided to hospitalized patients. Paper based documentation was in vogue and hence, the effects remained unclear. But, the study predicted that electronic documentation with day-to-day events would create a great impact on the quality of healthcare.

Nursing Information System (NIS) is a type of a Clinical Informatics System [37]. It is customized for nurses and has primarily two modules to assess the patient health and to document the care provided. The modules consist of pre-arranged menu-driven items which can be selected appropriately. The user interface is designed such that it is simple and resembles that of a paper based record. Front line nurses need knowledge at the point of care and EHRs should be able to provide them key insights, evidence and proper tools for optimal decision making and its implementation. Since nearly 50% of the healthcare workforce comprises of nurses, it is important to educate and train them about the technology, involved in EHR systems and making the best use of them. Informatics competence is necessary for seamless operation of digitalized healthcare system.

Future of EHRs and Beyond

Data is marking the borderline between the rich and deprived systems of healthcare. Analytics flourishes due to the advanced learning algorithms coupled with required computing infrastructure. Deep learning methods have tremendous potential to capture unnoticed insights from data. In a study of literature, it was found that deep learning techniques enhanced extraction of information, learning about the features, predicting traits and outcomes and the security of data [38].

Clinical Decision Support Systems(CDSS), Computerized Physician Order Entry (CPOE) and Precision Medicine require accurate data from EHRs to provide evidence based medicine and better quality of healthcare. On the contrary, the clinical notes that consist of narratives and key observations by clinicians have to be processed by Natural Language Processing (NLP) tools. While the clinical notes are not standardized, researchers are building customized NLPs in pursuit of understanding them.

Deep learning has brought out some latest, exciting, clinical applications such as adverse event prediction using EHR, targeted drug delivery, clinical research informatics, patient similarity assessment, prediction of readmission and stay duration, phenotyping and even integration with social networks[39]. EHR is a mine of data and it generates vast amount of 'big data'. Hence, the big data analytics on qualitative and quantitative data from EHRs can leverage improvements in the quality and performance of healthcare.

Smart gadgets are increasingly ubiquitous and leads to development of health applications based on the computing ability of the gadget. Further, Inter of Things (IoT) has enabled smart devices to capture data and transmit to clood servers or cloud platforms in which the computations are performed. A Sensor integration framework was proposed to integrate with

EHRs [40]. The framework collected vital signs and fitness activity-related data of subjects. The computation is performed over the edge of network and if necessary, is transmitted to the caregivers or physicians. This framework might be beneficial to include fitness activities into EHR data such that clinicians would get an overall health assessment.

ANALYSIS AND VISUALIZATION OF MEDICAL DATA

Medical data refers to any piece of detail associated with the patient. The data is usually collected by healthcare providers (or) researchers to keep track of the patient's health, identify the genes that influence the phenotype of an individual, find correlations to an unknown disease (or) to plan treatment [41]. The sources of medical data include EHR (Electronic Health Record), Administrative claim record, Clinical Registries, Prospective Cohort Studies, Clinical trials and Sensor data [42]. Clinical trials are conducted to identify effective drugs for the treatment of deadly diseases such as cancer. Prospective Cohort studies involve study of groups of individuals to determine the causal effect of various factors. Example includes study of factors that increases the risk of lung cancer in young men. Electronic Health Record (EHR) contain a wealth of information about patient health [43]. Figure 6 illustrates various types of patient- linked data.

Analyzing the medical data can yield information to support clinical decision, healthcare administration, mental and public health [44]. Medical Data Analysis can either be descriptive, predictive (or) prescriptive. Descriptive tasks offer a statistical viewpoint of the data. Given with the administrative claim record, it can help us identify the number of readmissions over a specific month. Predictive tasks unravel the hidden statistical information and predicts a possible outcome for the current data based on prior knowledge. It is highly useful in the context of diagnosis wherein the outcome of the diagnosis (infected with cancer) can be predicted from an x-ray image.Prescriptive analytics provides the best course of action for the possible outcome. The chapter is limited to techniques used for descriptive and predictive analytics.

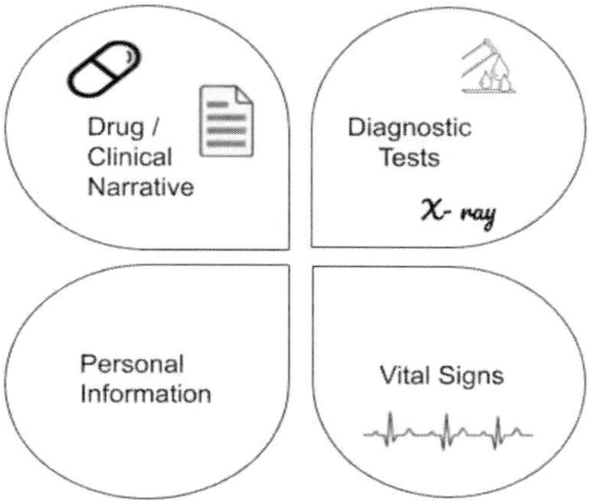

Figure 6. Pivotal Content in Electronic Health Record (EHR).

Data Processing Techniques

Medical data (or) Real world data (RWD) are maintained in multiple files and varied formats which poses huge challenge in deriving useful information. Raw Data is transformed into usable features through repetitive application of data preprocessing and feature engineering techniques. Data Visualization and Statistical procedures act as guiding tools to facilitate this transformation as shown in Figure 7.

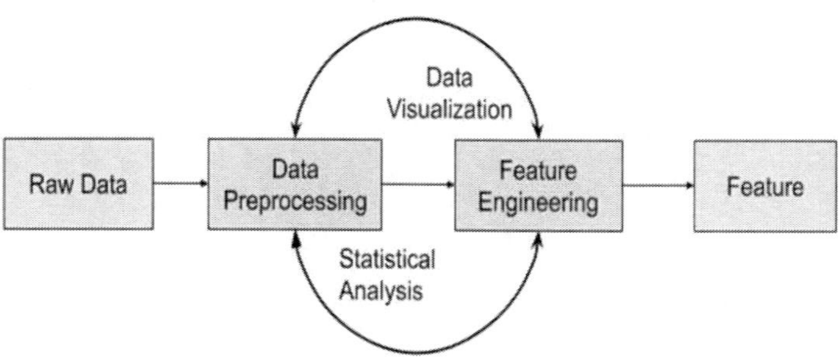

Figure 7. Data Processing Pipeline.

Data Preprocessing

The data obtained are often noisy, incomplete (or) inconsistent. Data preprocessing techniques are used to remove these inconsistencies in the data and convert it into a more suitable format to aid in clinical decision making. This section elaborates on state-of-art data preprocessing techniques.

Outlier Detection

Noise in the data may be attributed to manual error (or) system generated error. Presence of noise may affect the further statistical analysis. Either the feature (or) entire sample would be an outlier. To identify outliers for a specific feature, Z-score is used. It assumes a Gaussian distribution for the data and computes normalized feature using the following equation

$$Z_i = \frac{(X_i - \mu)}{\sigma} \quad (1)$$

where i denotes the sample

Here, μ and σ denotes the mean and the standard deviation of all the feature values (X_i). The feature values whose normalized value Z_i is greater than threshold $Z_{th}$are considered as outlier and are removed from the dataset. In a multidimensional space, where a sample point is represented by multiple features, Isolation Forest [6] is used to remove the outliers. The intuition behind the technique is to create decision trees by randomly splitting the data points on features with maximum information gain. Geometrically, decision trees partition the input data space based on arbitrary conditions over the features. If a data point is an outlier, then the point appears in lesser number of partitions and has a smaller path length as shown in Figure 8. The lines in Figure 8 indicate the partitions created in the data space. The outlier points occur only in a single partition, whereas other normal points occur in more than one partition.

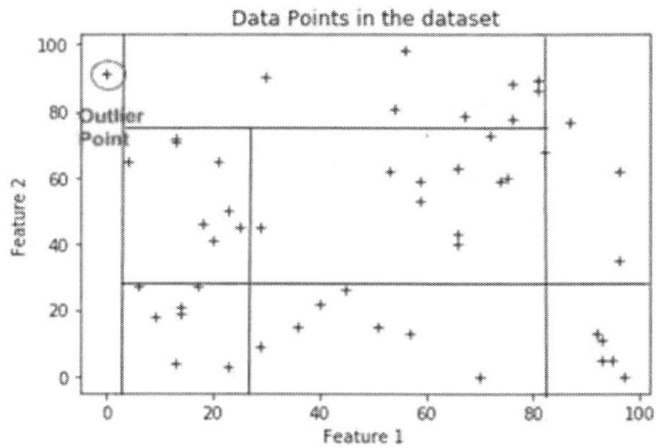

Figure 8. Partitions Created by Isolation Forest for random subset of points.

Missing Values

Missing Values are quite common in a medical dataset as the patients may have different profile and all data points do not have recorded values for all the features. The feature values may either have blank or NA (Not available) values. To address the missing values, following techniques are used.

1) Remove rows (data points) and columns (features) which has more than 75% of missing values.
2) Use Univariate Imputation to impute the missing values for a feature based on the inference over the same feature on the remaining set of data points. Mean, Median (or) Mode of the feature are common statistical values considered for replacement. For nominal attributes, missing values are replaced with most frequent label of the attribute.
3) Use Multivariate Imputation to impute the missing values for a feature using the regression model built on the remaining set of features. This imputation model reduces the noise introduced in the dataset during imputation by capturing the dependencies between the input features. For example, If the medication categorical attribute which takes two nominal values {yes (or) no} has a missing value for a data point, It would be appropriate to fill the

value based on illness feature rather than imputing it based on the frequency of labels.

Data Encoders

Categorical feature is more common in medical data but it cannot be ingested by machine learning algorithms directly. It is a normal convention to convert them into numerical features by encoding its labels. The popular techniques used are Ordinal Encoders, One Hot Encoders and Binary Encoders. Ordinal Encoders replace the label values with a numerical value based on the order of the labels in the dataset. One Hot Encoders creates features for every unique label of the categorical attribute where each feature either takes a value of 0 (or) 1. When there are many labels available for an attribute, one hot encoding rapidly increases the dimensionality of the input space. In such cases, Binary Encoding is used. It creates $log_2 n$ features and encodes the label values as unique binary strings of length $log_2 n$. Here, n denotes the number of unique values available for the categorical attribute. Usages of various encoders are shown in Table 5.

Table 5. Encoding categorical attribute tumor size

Data Points	Tumor Size	Ordinal Encoders	One Hot Encoders			Binary Encoders	
			F1	F2	F3	F1	F2
1	Small	1	1	0	0	0	0
2	High	2	0	1	0	0	1
3	Medium	3	0	0	1	1	0
4	Small	1	1	0	0	0	0
5	Medium	3	0	0	1	1	0

Like Categorical attributes, numerical attributes are also converted to derive meaningful inferences. For example, discretized version of age attribute could provide more information rather than using it directly. To transform numerical attribute into a categorical attribute, Discretization (or) Binarization are used.

1) Discretization divides the continuous attribute into specified number of bins. Popular Discretization methods include Equal Width Discretizer and Equal Frequency Discretizer. In Equal Width discretization, the complete range of the attribute is split into k categories of equal size. In Equal Frequency discretization, the range of the attribute is divided into k bins such that each bin contains the same frequency of elements. The value of k is determined by inspecting the frequency distribution of the attribute values.
2) Binarization is an extreme version of discretization with two bins. It converts the numerical attribute values into binary labels {0 or 1} by thresholding it. For instance, numerical blood pressure value can be converted into low (0) or high (1) by selecting a suitable threshold.

Feature Engineering

Not all the features could be useful in the construction of predictive models. Feature Engineering denotes the process of identification, selection (or) creation of the right set of features for the predictive task at hand.

1) Dimensionality Reduction - Most predictive models suffer from the curse of dimensionality. (i.e.,) when a system has a larger number of data points when compared to that of the number of features, predictive models fail. Projecting the data points onto a lower dimensional space with less number of features can resolve the problem. PCA (Principal Component Analysis) is the most widely used technique. It identifies orthogonal projection vectors which maximizes the variance of the data points (indicated using blue and green in Figure 9). Then, it transforms the data points onto the projection vectors. To reduce the dimension, only the

projection vectors which captures maximum variance are considered.

2) Feature Selection - Identifying subset of features which are more appropriate for the task. The two main categories include filter and wrapper methods.
   - Filter method uses statistical techniques to measure the correlation of every feature with respect to the task outcome. It helps in the identification of irrelevant features.
   - Wrapper method finds the best subset of features for the task through an iterative process of model construction. After every iteration, features are either added (or) removed based on the performance of the model. Common wrapper methods include
     - Forward Selection - It starts with an empty subset. After every iteration, new features are added to the subset until the performance of the model is not improved.
     - Backward Elimination - It starts with considering all the features. After every iteration, features are removed from the subset until the performance of the model is not improved.
     - Recursive Feature Elimination - It adopts a greedy optimization strategy to identify best subset of features. It identifies the best and the worst performing feature after every iteration and eliminates them. The method repeats the procedure until there are no features left in the set and ranks the feature in the order of elimination.

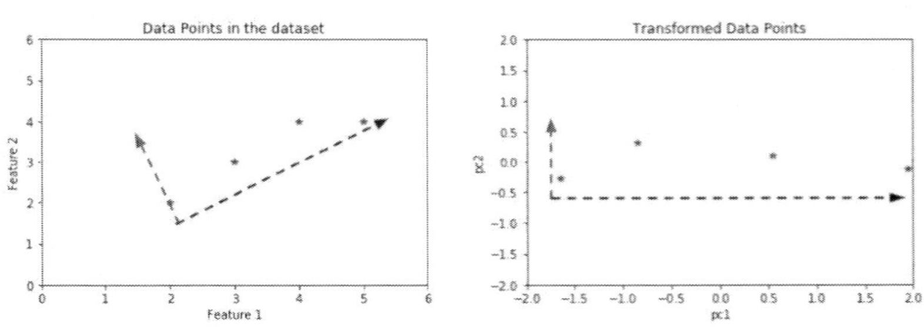

Figure 9. PCA Analysis.

1) Feature Construction - Creation of new features from the existing ones. It is done to ease the process of model construction. One such effective technique is feature crossing. It finds new feature by performing the cross between the available features. In certain situations, it converts even a non-linear data to linear data as shown in Figure 10. The plot on the left indicates a set of data points belonging to two different classes. Points are nonlinear in their own feature space as no linear classifier can separate them. When feature cross is applied, the features become separable as shown in the plot on the right.
2) Oversampling - Clinical data generally contains a large number of samples describing normal scenario and less number of samples for abnormal data.

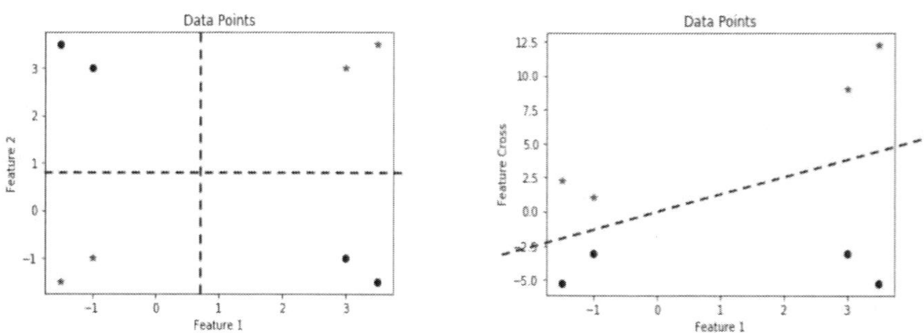

Figure 10. Addressing non -linearity through Feature Cross.

For example, Breast Wisconsin dataset [45] for breast pathology classification contains 357data points for benign class and 212data points for malignant class. This is known as class-imbalance problem. Any predictive model will be more sensitive to the target class with a large number of samples. This can be addressed by oversampling the minority class using SMOTE (Synthetic Minority Oversampling Technique). It creates new samples by changing the feature values randomly based on nearest neighbors.

1. Feature Scaling - When numerical features with varying range of values are present in the dataset, the predictive models will always be biased towards the feature with a larger range. Hence, it's a common practice to convert the feature values to a common scale. Min-Max normalization is the technique used to vary the scale of an attribute with range (MIN, MAX) to (NEW_MIN, NEW_MAX) using the following formula:

$$X_i = \frac{(X_i - min)}{(max - min)} * (new_{max} - new_{min}) + new_{min} \quad (2)$$

Data Exploration

To aid in the process of Feature engineering and Data preprocessing, data exploration is carried out. It depicts the underlying distribution of data using statistical techniques and data visualization.For the purpose of illustration, Breast Wisconsin Dataset [45] is used. It contains features extracted from the pathology image of the cancer patients. There are 589 instances and 32 features including a label denoting the malignancy level of the cancer.

Univariate Analysis

Histogram plot is an effective tool in understanding the central tendency (mean) and distribution (standard deviation) of continuous numeric attribute. It is used for inferring the probability distribution of a specific feature. Box plot provides a five number summary for the data including minimum, first quartile (25th percentile of the data), median, third quartile (75th percentile of the data) and maximum. Box plot serves as an effective tool in the identification of outliers. Any data point with a value greater than 1.5 * Inter quartile range (difference between first and third quartile) are considered as outliers. Figure 11 shows the histogram and box plot constructed for the feature radius_mean.

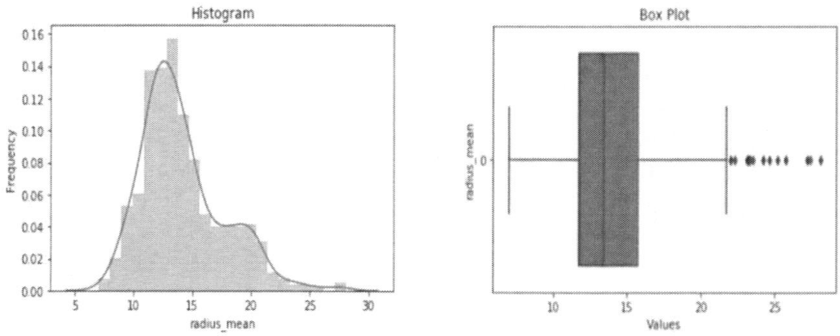

Figure 11. Interpreting radius_mean using Histogram and Box Plot.

Histogram plot shows the distribution along with the kernel density estimation which approximates the frequency distribution. From the graph, it is evident that the feature follows normal distribution. Similarly, Box plot offers a five number summary and indicates the presence of outliers which are shown as points extending the whisker at value of 22.

Bar chart is used for categorical attributes to infer the frequency of each label associated with the attribute. It will be helpful in understanding the minority class labels.

BIVARIATE ANALYSIS

During analysis, it is always required to ascertain the relationship between multiple features and also between the feature and the response variable. Scatter plot brings out the associations between numerical attributes by interpreting feature values as data points on two dimensional Cartesian plane.

It depicts the correlation between various features which helps in identification and removal of the redundant features. Correlation captures the linear relation between the attributes. In Figure 12, the second plot represents the set of features which are linearly dependent on each other (i.e.,) when the value of one feature increases, the other feature also increases whereas in the first plot, features are linearly independent.

Statistically, Pearson Correlation Coefficient is used to find the strength of association between two numerical attributes X1 and X2. It is computed using the following formula:

$$\rho_{X1,X2} = \frac{COV(X1,X2)}{\sigma_{x1}\sigma_{x2}} \quad (3)$$

Where $COV(X1,X2) = \frac{\sum_{i=1}^{n}(x1-\bar{x1})(x2-\bar{x2})}{n}$ (4)

Here, n denotes the number of samples, $\bar{x1}$ and $\bar{x2}$ indicate the mean of the attributes x1 and x2 respectively and σ_{x1} and σ_{x2} represent the standard deviation of the features. The value of ρ lies in the range between -1 and +1. -1 implies negative correlation, +1 implies positive correlation and zero indicates no correlation. Heat map is an effective visualization tool used to represent the correlation between all pairs of numerical attributes in the dataset. It depicts the values in a matrix of size n*n where n denotes the number of attributes. Values are encoded using colors which differ with the strength of association. Lighter shade indicates positive correlation and Darker shade indicate negative correlation. Redundant set of features can easily be identified from this plot. The features 'radius_mean', 'area_mean' and 'perimeter_mean' exhibit strong association which is very evident from the Figure 13.

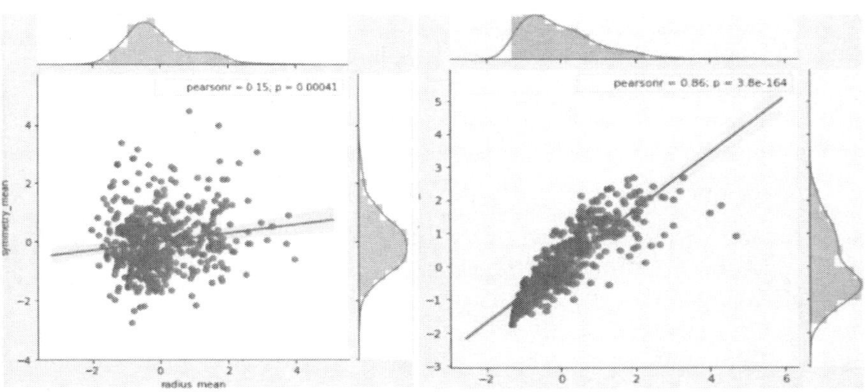

Figure 12. Scatter plot between features.

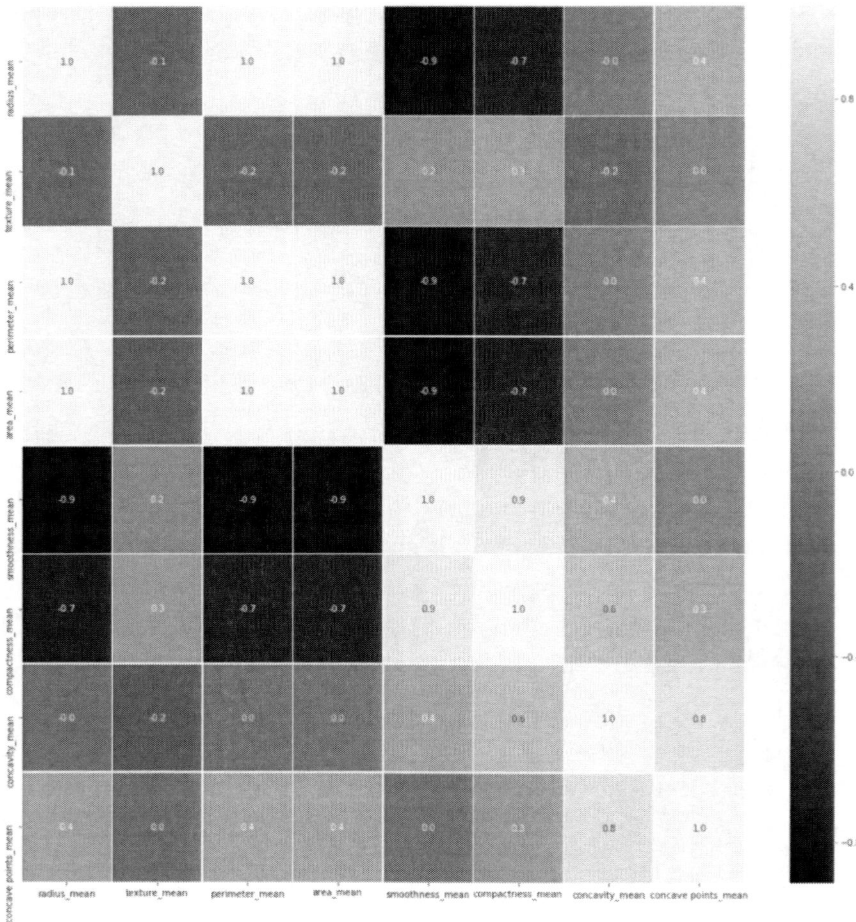

Figure 13. Heat Map for subset of features in the dataset.

Pair - plot is an extension of scatter plot; where correlations between more than two parameters are depicted. It finds scatter plot between every pair of parameters and displays the same in the form of a matrix as shown in Figure 14. These plots are highly useful in validating the linear correlation between the subset of features.

To find the correlation between two categorical attributes, chi square test is used. It accumulates the difference between expected frequencies and actual frequencies for every unique combination of attributes. It returns a probability based on the computed sum and the number of samples. A probability of zero indicates strong correlation and a value of 1 indicates that the attributes are linearly independent.

$$\chi^2 = \sum_{i=1}^{r} \frac{\sum_{j=1}^{c}(n_{ij}-e_{ij})^2}{e_{ij}} \text{where } e_{ij} = \frac{n_i n_j}{n} \quad (5)$$

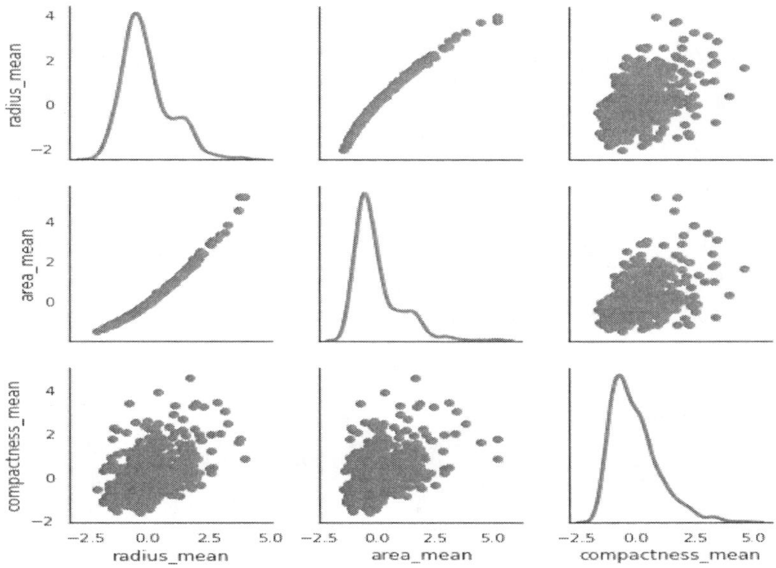

Figure 14. Pair plot between set of features.

Here, e_{ij}represent the expected frequency of the label i for the first feature and label j for the second feature. n_{ij}represent the observed frequency of labels i and j for the first and second feature respectively. Unique label values of the attributes are indicated by r and c respectively. Graphically, stacked column chart is used to capture the dependency between the categorical attributes. It captures the percentage of samples for each unique label of an attribute with respect to all the labels of the other attributes as shown in Figure 15.

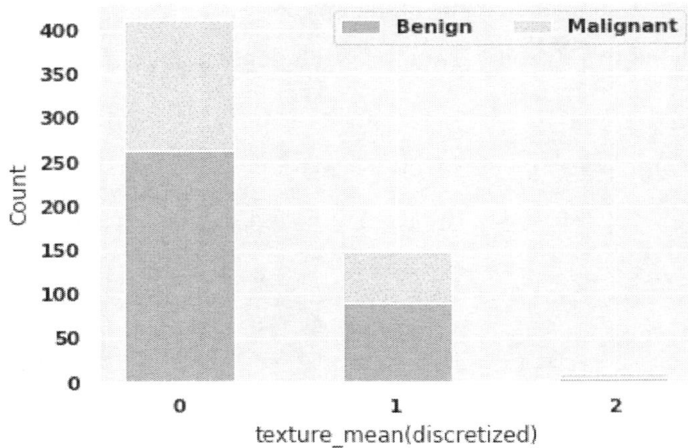

Figure 15. Malignancy-wise Distribution of texture_mean Categories.

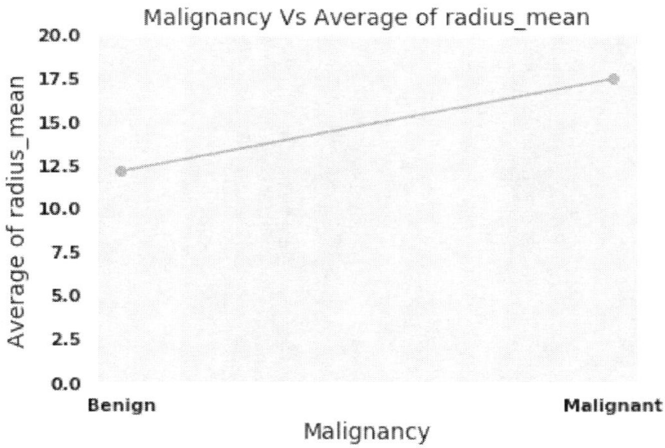

Figure 16. Line Chart.

To understand and assess the association between a categorical attribute and a numerical attribute, ANOVA (Analysis of Variance) is performed. It provides statistical analysis of whether the groups of the categorical attribute are different from each other based on the numerical attribute. It computes the mean square difference between the groups and within the groups. Further, uses the measures to compute Fisher Discriminant ratio $F = MS_B/MS_W$ and compares it with critical significance value α.If the value of F is found to be greater than αvalue, then the groups are found to be statistically different. A line chart is used to depict the difference in the average of numerical attribute with respect to the categorical attribute as shown in Figure 16.

Tools for Visualization

There is a plethora of tools in the market to support the data visualization. This section reviews the popular open-source software's and packages. Plotly is a general use visualization tool. It supports integration with languages such as python. It allows users to setup an account and store all the charts within the account. It also provides options for organizing the charts and creating multi-chart visualization. Tableau Public is open-source version of Tableau; widely used tool in the Business Intelligence community. It enables a user to combine the charts into single piece of content through interactive dashboards and infographics.D3.js is a JavaScript library which offers support for powerful visualization. The library is so massive and has options for every possible thing that can be done with graphs. The examples at d3.js gallery [46] serves as a testimony of package's humongous capabilities. Chart.js is a minimalistic package which supports basic plotting. Two widely used languages for business analytics: python and R has support for data visualizations through its libraries and packages. In python, the packages matplotliband seaborn can be leveraged upon for creating basic and sophisticated plots.

Healthcare Data Analytics

In today's world, with every transaction and process digitized, there is a vast amount of data generated from different organizations in the world. Using big data analytic techniques, these companies can gain various insights to identify the loss points and streamline their operations. The same goes for health-care industry as well. These data analytic techniques are capable of handling vast amount of dataHealth care data analytics is the process of collecting and analyzing data from various sources with a view to obtain insights and aid in decision making process in the health-care industry. This helps in providing best care to the patients at the lowest cost as well as stream-lining the operations in a hospital.For this purpose, health-care data analytics is used in both macro and micro levels of the health-care industry. The collection of data is vital. It ranges from the cost incurred to function the facility to the vital signs of the patient. Each category of data has to be collected and analyzed appropriately to ensure true and precise insights are provided to the concerned personnel. With the aid of visual data, key-decision makers will be able to explore the performance gaps and take the right course of actions to address them.

The recent trend in the health care industry suggests a shift from service-based approach to a value based care model. This shift has resulted in giving more emphasis to improving the range of services provided and the efficiency of these services. In this scenario, data analytics play a crucial role to ensure that right decisions are taken at the right time. This can be a change in the course of treatment of a patient or an additional investment in the medical research to cutting down the daily cost of operations as depicted in Figure 17. The data trend aids in visualizing the pitfalls and opportunities in real-time.

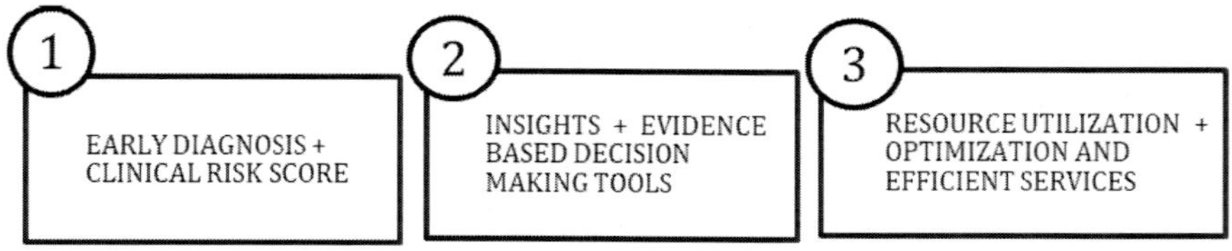

Figure 17. Benefits of a Data Analytic Tool in Healthcare Systems.

The health care data analytics is implemented with the help of embedded solutions. This offers the required level of security and connectivity. The majority of patient health records are hence digitized these days. This helps in identification of patient history and patterns more efficient. High-risk patients benefit from these services the most since the health care providers has an opportunity to intervene and reduce their emergency visits to the hospitals by taking appropriate corrective strategies. These patients require continuous monitoring. The growth of Internet-of-Things has helped in providing solutions to ensure that these patients are monitored remotely as well. The care and attention the high-risk patients require cannot be provided unless sufficient data is provided to the medical fraternity.

Many mishaps occurring in the health care industry can be directly attributed to errors from human intervention, such as, a doctor might prescribe the wrong medication or the wrong dosage to a patient. There is a higher probability of such occurrences, especially, when the concerned personnel is overloaded. A BI platform can be programmed to continuously analyze the patient data including patient history and current condition and prescribe medication accordingly. Also, this software can be enabled to alert the concerned personnel of unusual prescriptions or dosages. This ensures that the errors occurring due to human intervention are limited to a minimum. Also, it serves to check that the unfortunate incidences occurring towards the patient.

The crowding of emergency rooms or auxiliary services like laboratories, X-Ray Departments, Oncology Rooms etc., is one of the most common problems faced by a health care institution that leads to many serious complications. This situation proves to be a hindrance for the patient to get effective and efficient treatment [47]. Poor handling of resources, under-staffing and competency issues of the employed staff are two main reasons for such a scenario. With the help of a BI, the decision makers would be provided with the information or alert regarding such a scenario before it happens. Such small changes are more or less like pre-emptive strikes. The changes though small in nature have results of great magnitude. The data analytic tools assist not only in devising strategies for current issues, it also serves to provide information regarding problems that may arise in the future. Such tools filter massive amounts of patient history and patters data in seconds. This helps the physicians to formulate the best course of treatment to a patient. The potential of data analytic tools in diagnosis of diseases are limitless. These include

- Epidemic prediction

- Disease cures.
- Quality of life improvement.
- Preventable care.
- Early detection.
- eRisk assessment.

The hospitals have to invest a huge amount of money for its daily operation. Staff Remunerations and Energy Bills incur a huge amount between themselves. With the help of a BI, the hospital management can easily get visual data of their current staffing requirement, whether it is in correlation with the admission rates, and the major areas in which energy is being consumed. This identification will help to bring down the daily cost of operation thus directly resulting in huge financial savings.

The health-care data analytics works in4 stages. These are

- Descriptive Analytics
- Diagnostic Analytics
- Predictive Analytics
- Prescriptive Analytics

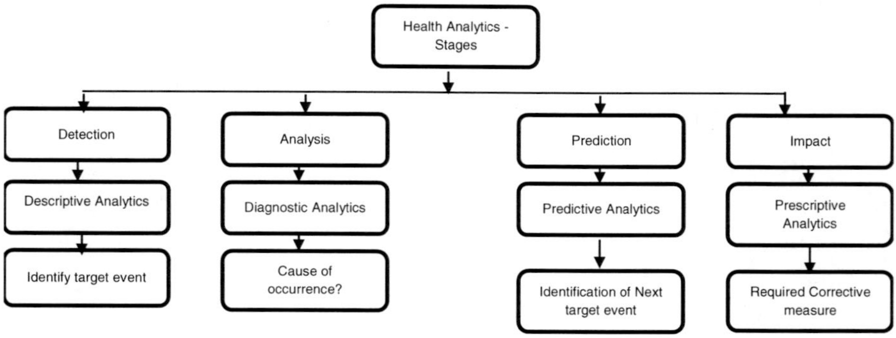

Figure 18. Stages of Health-Care Analytics.

A block diagram of different stages of health care analytics is as shown in Figure 18.Descriptive Analytics deal with the data related to the events that have already happened. This helps to answer questions like total number of admissions over a month, average number of X-Rays taken in a week etc. [48].These types of questions can be answered with the help of historical data and simple statistical tools like total, percentages, mean and standard deviation. When tracked for over a certain period of time, the descriptive analytical tools help to see if a certain course of action is meeting the intended goal.

Diagnostic Analytics works on answering the question of "Why it happened." With the help of data collected and extensive research and analysis on it with the help of statistical tools and visualizing techniques, the root cause of the problem under concern is identified and addressed. For example, a higher length of stay at the MRI – service can be attributed to either incompetent operator, faulty machine or any other problem. A Root-Cause-Analysis, when done, will let the decision makers take the corrective actions appropriately.

Predictive Analytic tools aids to understand what will happen or as the name suggest, predict the future with respect to a context. It utilizes the historical data along with the corrective measure taken to evaluate the probability of a target event occurring in the future. While making a "future prediction," it takes into account the hidden patterns in the raw data and then extrapolating it make the prediction [47].

Prescriptive Analytics aids in deciding the right course of action to overcome or totally avoid problems that may occur in the future. It can be said that it answers the question "What can be done about that?" based on the results of predictive analytics. For e.g., If a patient is found to be in high risk category for a certain type of cancer, the concerned doctor can take necessary course of action to ensure he is completely avoiding that risk or starting him on right course of treatment so that it can be kept in check and cleared. To obtain such insights, prescriptive analytics uses complex tools, machine learning algorithms, business tents and a huge data set. Healthcare industry benefits significantly by employing prescriptive analytics for its streamlining.

There are a lot of analytic tools that can improve health-care industry. Depending upon the results that are to be obtained, appropriate tool has to be chosen. Each tool differs in the insight it offers or the question it answers. The descriptive and diagnostic analytics have a more reactive approach while the predictive and prescriptive analytics are proactive in nature. The complexity to implement also varies a lot. Descriptive analytics being the simplest and prescriptive being the most complex.

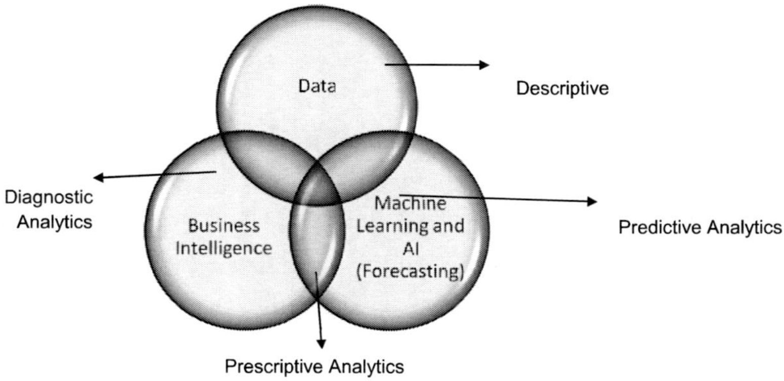

Figure 19. A Venn diagram depicting the relationship between Data, Business Intelligence and Machine learning for each type of analytic solution.

The Venn diagram shown in Figure 19 depicts how data, business intelligence and Machine learning or AI systems are related to make each type analytic technique. As stated previously, the descriptive analytics give insight to the events that have already occurred. It works with raw data and simple statistical tools to provide quantitative values to the analyst. A combination of raw data and business intelligence is utilized by diagnostic analytic techniques to conduct Root-Cause-Analysis and problems of such kind. The Predictive Analytic technique uses the results from both descriptive and diagnostic analytic techniques to shed light on hidden patterns in the data and predict future target events. Once the target events have been predicted, to maximize or minimize its probability of occurrence, the prescriptive analytic techniques use all three quantities and suggest multiple course-of-actions.

Exploratory Data analytics takes a different approach. In this technique emphasis is given to fully understand the data before it is fed to machine learning and artificial intelligence systems. It relies heavily on visual aids to shed light on important parameters and variables and trends or pattern within the data set.

Descriptive Analytics

Descriptive analytics is the most basic and simple of the four different types of analytical tools. It ensures that the data collected is sourced properly and is presented well i.e., data itself is not changed during the process of collecting it. Insights into the process or operation are gained with the help of score cards, bar charts, cluster analysis and pie-diagrams. Simple statistical tools like percentages, mean and standard deviation are used to obtain the quantitative representation. Since the collection of data itself will act as the foundation on which the analysis and decisions are based upon, the collection process is given utmost importance. With the help of visual aids and quantitative values, the descriptive analytics enables the stake holders gain perspective and interpret information regarding the operation or business.

Descriptive analytic tools have a more data-driven approach when compared to the other models. A large number of organizations in the healthcare industry rely on with descriptive analytics to understand past and current trend regarding the quality of patient care and then make informed decisions. Descriptive analytic models provide insights using visual aids for easy understanding of the current scenario in a particular entity. The raw data collected from various sources are categorized, characterized, aggregated and classified before to obtain the necessary information. [48]. The visual aids used to summarize the insights might be in the form of meaningful charts and reports that, for example, illustrate patient hospitalizations, physician performance, utilization management, and the like [48]. The descriptive analytics is based on the collected data and no kind of assumptions are made at this level.

The descriptive analytics, in a broad sense, will help us to answer the questions of following type:

- Number of Out-Patients
- Number of Admissions
- Average Number of Discharges in a day
- Number of Staff/Patient

Descriptive analytic tools, typically, generate various reports using which different healthcare decisions and their implications on services performance, clinical outcomes and results can be studied [48]. The organizations are therefore equipped to make informed and effectual decisions to manage real-time, or near real time data, what can be called operational content, and capture all patients' visual data. This aids to illuminate hidden patterns among patients, for example, patterns related to hospital re-admissions, stream-lining of hospital operations for a better bottom-line. [49].

Descriptive analytics is the simplest technique that provides an insight into the big data collected from different points of the operation of an institution. It serves the summary of the data collected in the most readable format. No assumptions are made. The insight thus served is utilized by superior data analytic techniques to understand why a particular event occurred and what the future is.The current scenario or status of operation of an organization is understood with the help of the data presented. The analysts use this summary as a tool to identify patterns and trends that have occurred in the past.

The commonly tools to analyze the big data are as listed below:

- Assessing Correlation
- Univariate Statistical Inference
- Multivariate Statistical Inference
- Hierarchical Cluster Analyses

Assessing Correlations

Using this technique, the extent to which two variables are related is measured. This value will vary from +1 to -1. A visual depiction is as shown in Figure 20. If the value is closer to plus or minus 1, then it is said to suggest a higher degree of correlation.

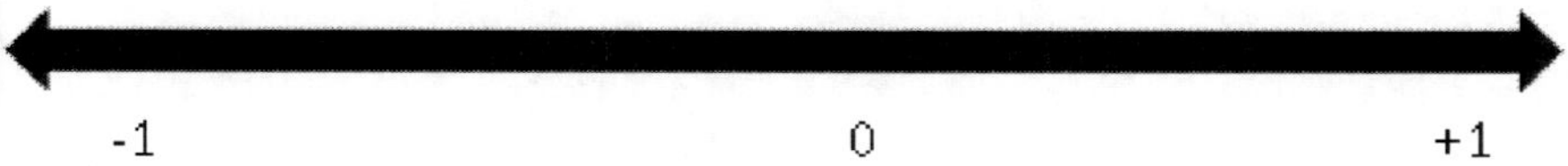

Figure 20. Range of Coefficient of Correlation.

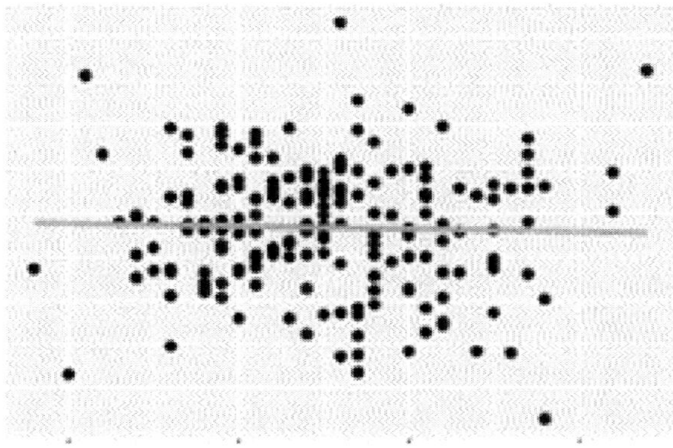

Figure 21(a). Weak Correlation.

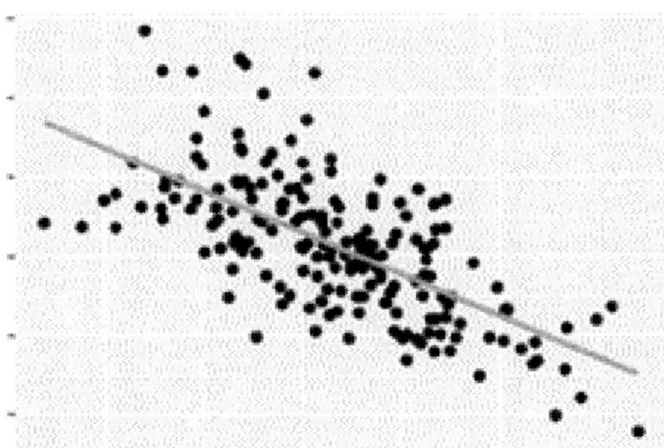

Figure 21(b). Moderately Negative Correlation.

On the other hand, if this value is closer to 0, then a weaker relation is said to exist between the two variables under consideration. Often, a scatter-plot is used to obtain the visual representation of the collected data.

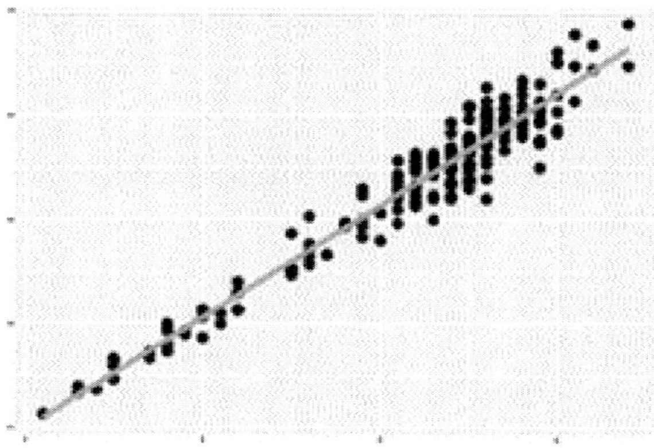

Figure 21(c). Strongly Positive Correlation.

Graphs shown in Figures 21(a), 21(b) and 21(c) show the different correlations between two variables.There exists another technique known as partial correlation which is widely used in big data analytics. It not only computes the correlation between two variables, but also finds out the direction of their correlation. In this technique one more variable is taken into consideration. This variable is called the covariate and has will have significant effect on the strength of correlation between the two variables under consideration. These techniques are highly popular in tracking the performance of athletes and sportsmen. It is use to identify their strength and weaknesses in their game, improve reaction time and stamina. Also, they are extensively employed to find out correlations between game-time and extent of injuries to these players. Injuries like Ligament tear on ankles, knees and shoulder joints are career-ending. These tools now serve the purpose to help the physicians understand when the player is approaching a burn-out condition and manage his fitness regimen or game-time appropriately.

Hierarchical Clustering

There are two main types of hierarchical clustering algorithms namely Agglomerative and Divisive. In the agglomerative method, a bottom-up approach is taken. Individual elements are considered as a cluster initially. With each iteration, two clusters that are most similar, is combined to form a bigger cluster. This process is continued until elements are a part of single cluster. The divisive method is exactly the reverse of this approach. It starts by considering all elements to be a part of a one cluster. With each iteration the two most dissimilar clusters are separated and the process continues until all individual elements exist as single element clusters. The process is as shown in Figure 22.

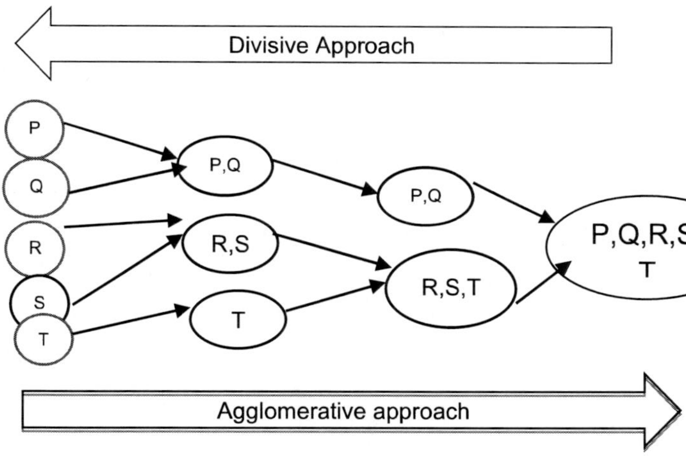

Figure 22. Different approaches for Hierarchical Clustering.

The measure of correlation between two clusters is taken as the distance or dissimilarity between them. This value can be obtained with the help of following techniques:

- Maximum linkage clustering: In this technique, the dissimilarities between elements of 2 clusters are computed. This process is then repeated for the entirety of both the clusters. The largest distance between the elements of two clusters is taken as the measure or extent of dissimilarity. This technique results in compact clusters.
- Minimum linkage clustering: The approach in this technique is similar to that of Maximum Linkage Clustering. It differs in the fact that instead of taking the largest distance between the elements of two clusters, smallest distance is considered. This is considered

as the measure of correlation between the two clusters. The clusters tend to have spread-out nature because of loose linkages between the elements of two clusters under consideration.

- Average linkage clustering: The dissimilarities between elements of 2 clusters are computed. The mean of all the dissimilarities thus obtained is taken as the distance between two clusters
- Centroid Linkage clustering: in this technique, the centroid for both the clusters are calculated. The dissimilarity between the two clusters is taken as the distance between these two centroids.

Those personnel who engage in descriptive analytics generate reports shed light on events that have already occurred, resources that have been consumed, or patients who have a new diagnosis on their charts [48].This helps to identify the number of patients living with diabetes, benchmark outcomes against government expectations, or identify areas for improvement on clinical quality measures or other aspects of care [48].

Diagnostic Analytics

Diagnostic Analytic tools help to understand "Why something is happening? "or "Why did it happen?." It is based on the results of descriptive analytics.Diagnostic Analytic tools employ techniques such as drill-down, data discovery, data mining and correlations to give useful insights to the users. They help to identify and answer those questions which cannot be answered by just viewing the data. Such anomalies are identified by exploring patterns outside the data sets. The causal nature of these occurrences has to be determined and correlated to the variables in the existing data sets. Probability theory, regression analysis, filtering, and time-series data analytics are also used for shedding light on such hidden correlations within the dataset.

Previously, these calculations and research were done by analysts and the efficiency of the process varied a lot from one analyst to the other. With the help of machine learning techniques and artificial intelligence, we are able to enable computing machines augment highly efficient data analysts. These machines are highly effectual at recognizing patterns, detecting anomalies and surfacing 'unusual' events [50]. Diagnostic analytics also ensures that unintentional bias and misinterpretation of correlation as causation is reduced to the minimum.

Some example scenario where diagnostic analytics could be applied are

- Why has there been a dip in X-Ray facility usage
- Why did the people visit hospital last week?
- Why has there been an increase in the usage of MRI facility

These questions are inherently based on the results of descriptive analytics. It has identified an increase or decrease in the usage or visits. Diagnostic analytics try to answer why that change happened. It factors in staff efficiency, staff/patient, number, efficiency and effectiveness of laboratory resources and cost of each service. All these parameters together with the results from the descriptive analytics help the analysts to find out patterns and correlations.

Different tools are available to implement diagnostic data analytics and most of them are also used to implement the descriptive data analytics. Often K-means Cluster Analysis is used diagnostic data analytics. Clustering is defined as the process of identifying and grouping similar set of elements or observations within a data set. Thus, each cluster of observation will be dissimilar and easy to identify and interpret. K-means clustering, as the name suggests, splits the data set into k-groups. The main requirement in this process is that the data set is normalized. This normalization ensures that two variables are comparable, mean becomes zero and the standard deviation becomes one [51]. Also, no missing data should exist in the data set. If at all there is any data missing, that data should also be estimated and normalized.

The classification of data is done by estimating the dissimilarity or distance of observations between two clusters. Each cluster is identified by its centroid or the mean of all observations included in that cluster. The value for 'k' is pre-defined by the analyst.

The dissimilarity between two clusters is quantified by comparing their distance measures. The classical methods for distance measures are*Euclidean*and*Manhattan distances*, which are defined as follow:

Euclidean distance:

$$d_{euc}(x,y)=\sqrt{\sum_{i=1}^{n}(x_i - y_i)^2} \quad (6)$$

Manhattan distance:

$$d_{man}(x,y)=\sqrt{\sum_{i=1}^{n}(x_i - y_i)} \quad (7)$$

Where, *x*and*y*are two vectors of length*n*. Though, there are various methods to calculate the distance, the choice of method depends on the type of question that has to be answered. Euclidean method is the most often preferred. The main objective of this approach is to minimize the total variation within a cluster. Among the several k-means algorithms, Hartigan-Wong algorithm is commonly used. It defines the total within-cluster variation as the sum of squared distances Euclidean distances between items and the corresponding centroid:

$$W(C_k)=\sum(x_i - \mu_k)^2 \quad (8)$$

Where $x_i$is a data point belonging to the clusterC_k and $\mu_k$is the mean value of the points assigned to the clusterC_k. Priority is given to minimize the total sum of squares variation within the cluster. This directly translates to the compactness of the cluster.

This approach has a disadvantage that the number of clusters has to be pre-specified. Also, this approach is sensitive to the ordering of the data. Any change in the ordering can directly affect the results generated.

Predictive Analytics

Once the and why have been identified and addressed, the next step is to analyze the data to see if a pattern emerges. This helps in predicting the occurrences of certain events and results of drug trials etc. Predictive analytics is capable of quantifying the risk factor and find relationships in health data. This cannot be achieved with descriptive and diagnostic analytics alone or together. The data set is huge and advanced techniques are required to implement predictive analytics. Data mining and pattern recognition algorithms assist to detect hidden patterns in the huge data segments. These may be

- Which patients may be under high risk category in the next quarter?
- Will there be an increase in number of admissions, if so, is there a higher staff requirement?
- Will there be a higher usage of laboratory facilities?

In predictive analytics, historical data is used to train models. It can then predict future events by employing advanced computational techniques such as machine learning [52].The data set used for predictive analytics is huge. The tools are utilized to identify pattern and predict which patient is more at risk. This helps to prioritize and provide the necessary attention and care to those who are in urgent need of it. Although, the predictive analytic tools are able to aid us in identifying the risk patients, it cannot prevent adverse events such as hospitalization. That being said, the predictive analytics is an important tool for the health-care industry as it helps them prepare better for future target events.

Predictive analytics utilize the results of descriptive and diagnostic data analytics to uncover the hidden patters or trends. This revelation helps in predicting what may happen in the future. To make such inferences from the past data, tools like linear regression, time series forecasting, multiple data modeling and simulation techniques are used.Some of the popular machine learning based approach is as listed below:

- Naïve Bayes Classifier
- Linear Regression
- Linear Model Selection
- Support Vector Machines

Naïve Bayes Classifier

This technique or approach is one of the simplest probabilistic classifiers used in predictive data analytics. When compared to the advanced and complex approaches, this approach is inferior in its accuracy and classification abilities. Nonetheless, with the help of its grounded assumptions and naïve design, it out performs the more superior techniques with its quickness to solve many complex real-world problems.

It is based on Bayes theorem and is built on the concept of conditional probability. The formula for calculating probability is

$$P(A/X) = \{P(A) \, . \, P(X/A)\}/P(X) \tag{9}$$

Where P(A) is the probability of the outcome from the historical data obtained previously, P(X) is the probability of predictor variables and P(X|A) is the likelihood. i.e., the probability of observing the predictor values. In layman terms, it can be expressed as [51],

Probability of an event happening = (Prior occurrences x Likelihood) / (Evidence obtained from data)

Usually, if there are Z classes and p variables, then it requires Z^p computations in total to complete the process. The classifier inherently assumes that one independent of another. This approach enables the computation to be scaled further if required. Also, since the target events are assumed to be mutually independent of each other, the total number of computations to obtain the probability of a target even in the future is considerably reduced to (Z x p) computations.

The simplistic nature of this approach is its handicap as well. For e.g., if there is no history of a particular target event available in the historical data collected, the classifier will give the probability of that event happening in the future as zero.

i.e., $P(A|X) = 0$

To overcome this hindrance, a *Laplace Smoother* [51] is used. It ensures that all target events, even if there it has no occurrences in the history, will generate non-zero probabilistic value.

Linear Regression

It is one of the simplest models available that utilizes a supervised learning approach. Linear regression is one of the best tools, though old, that can be used to predict the quantitative response of a system. In this approach, a predictive relationship is first formulated from the data set collected. Then using a test set, it is then checked for validity and strength of these relationships. To formulate the predictive relationship, a training data set is used. In its crude form, a linear regression analysis will predict the quantitative response of a system on the basis of a single predictor variable. For eg, to predict whether a person is susceptible to a particular disease depending on his age and the calorie he consumes in a day, this approach assumes a linear relationship between the variables.

Support Vector Machines

The rapid development in computing and information technology greatly affected the statistical modeling techniques. With this advent came the supportvector machines. This approach takes in classes of observations made available from the results of descriptive data analytic techniques. From these classes of observations, the support vector machines construct boundaries so as to predict which future target event will belong to which group of observations based on their measurements. The support vector machines are capable of handling any number of classes, observations and dimensions [9]. It is not confined to any state and has great flexibility to be used in any classification or identification application.

The boundary of a class in SVM is identified with the help of Maximal Margin Classifier. The objective of this classifier is to identify that linear boundary which maximizes the total distance between the line and the closes point in each class. Such a scenario rarely appears while solving real-world problems. In such cases a modified approach, known as Support Vector Classifiers, is used. In this approach, the boundary of each class is not as well defined as the Maximal Margin Classifier approach. Also, there are possible occurrences of class overlap are also there. These classifiers are actually a subset of SVM. Support Vector Machines can construct classification boundaries that are nonlinear in shape [51].

As healthcare organizations are continuously trying to achieve better care coordination and improve patient care outcomes, they are quick to rely upon predictive analytic tools. According to a 2017 study by the Society of Actuaries, 93 percent of health organizations say predictive analytics is important to the future of their business, with 89 percent of providers currently using predictive analytics or planning to do so in the next five years [53].An artificial intelligence algorithm CheXNeXt, developed by researchers at Stanford University, uses predictive analytics in imaging to screen chest X-rays in a matter of seconds to detect 14 different pathologies with high accuracy [53].

Prescriptive Diagnostics

Prescriptive Diagnostics tries to find out the answers to the problems posed by predictive analytics. It takes predictive analytics to a higher level by suggesting what may be the course of action to avoid or ensure target events.Prescriptive analytics abets in quantifying the effect of future decisions. This aids in analyzing possible outcomes before the decisions are actually made. At its best, prescriptive analytic tools will be able to predict, not only if a target event will happen, but also why it will happen. With this information, it will provide recommendations for required actions to the decision makers. This helps to take advantage of the predictions [54]. For example, if the predictive diagnostics points out to a larger influx of admissions, the prescriptive analytics will help to indicate what strength of staff might be required to impart effective care to all of them. It basically uses results obtained from all the three previous analytic techniques.

Prescriptive analytics suggest intervention at the right stage and right time so that, the bottom line of a health-care institution is bettered, its operation is stream-lined and it is prepared for future adverse events in the most efficient manner. The multiple futures predicted by prescriptive analytic technique is based on big data, machine learning algorithms, real-time feed, historical and transactional data and multiple computational modeling procedures.

The tools or approaches used by the predictive and prescriptive analytic techniques are quite the same. Some of the commonly preferred approaches are as listed below,

- Regression Trees
- Random Forests
- Gradient Boosting Machines

Regression Trees

Regression trees split the data set into several smaller groups. Then a constant is set for each such group. With the help of subgroups, a definitive model for prescriptive data analytics can be built as shown in Figure 23. Bootstrapping or aggregating these subgroups serves to improve the efficiency and quickness of the technique. Also, the regression tree approach acts as the foundation on which random forests and gradient boosting machines are built.

The subgroups are created on the basis of Classification and Regression Tree. The subgroups are formed by recursive portioning of the original observation set and a constant is provided for each such set. The constant provided to a subgroup is decided by the average response values of all the observations in that group.

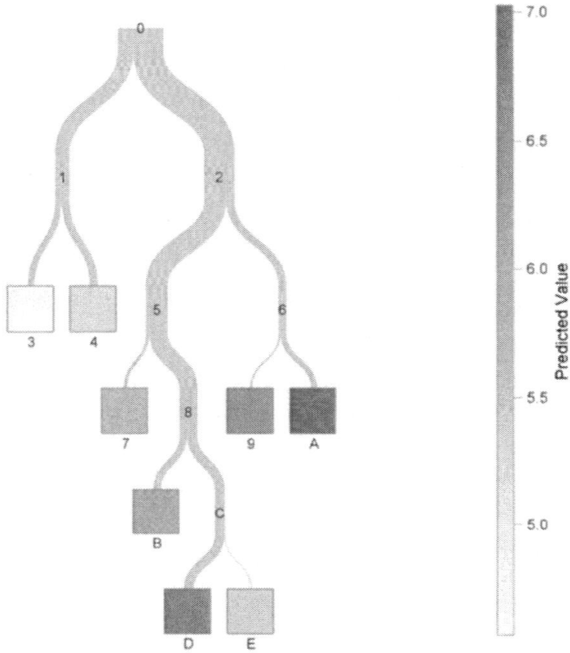

Figure 23. Regression Tree.

To generalize, if we consider a system with a continuous response variable Z and input variables $x_1, x_2 \ldots x_n$, then

$$Z = f\ (x) = \sum C_i I(X_{1,}, X_{2,} X_{3,} X_{4,} \ldots \ldots \ldots X_{n,}) R_j$$

where R_i is the region for constant C_i. In this approach, the partition of variables is implemented in a top-down manner. At first the entirety of the data set *S*, is considered. A search is conducted for each distinct value of all the input variables to find the predictor and the split value. Only then, the data set S is partitioned into two regions (R_1andR_2) such that the overall sums of squares error are minimized [51]:

$$minimize\{Sum\ of\ Squares\ Error\} = \{\textstyle\sum_{i\epsilon R_1} (y_1 - c_1)^2 \mp \sum_{i\epsilon R_2} (y_i - c_2)^2\} \qquad (10)$$

In the next step, the 2 regions formed previously will be again split into two. The process continues until, a stopping condition comes true. This process has the disadvantage that it has poor performance on unseen data or conditions. To overcome the overfitting phenomenon of a deep and complex tree, proper biasing is required at the lower level subgroups. This will result in a prediction of stable and accurate results as well as it will be enabled to generalize the unseen conditions or data. The main advantage of the regression tree approach is that it is very easy to interpret. The important variables in making the prediction can be easily identified. Even if complete data is not provided, it is still possible to obtain a valid result.

Random Forests

Random Forest approach is a modified regression tree and bagging approach. In this technique the high variance and poor performance of a single tree structure is addressed. Here a large number of decorrelated trees are formed. The main difference of random forest approach from that of regression is that a random component is introduced during the process of building a tree. The introduction of this component significantly reduces the variance in overall prediction and improves its performance. Such trees are not completely independent since the original predictors still influence every split in each iteration. This phenomenon is known as tree correlation. To reduce the variance, the strength of correlation between two trees must be minimized. This is obtained with the help of random component mentioned previously.

This component is introduced in two ways [51],

1) Bootstrap: It is very much similar to bagging. Here, each tree is grown to a bootstrap resampled data set. This makes no two trees the same. Thus resulting in a decorrelated structure.
2) Split-variable randomization: During each partition, a split variable has to be found. The search for the split variable is limited to a random subset of$m$of the$p$variables. In regression tree approach, typical default values are used. This can be considered only as a

tuning parameter. When, the randomization process amounts to using only step 1 it takes the same structure as bagging.

The random forest approach has good performance. It includes a set of built-in validation data. Thus a sacrifice of data for extra validation is not required. Also, no kind of pre-processing of data is required in this technique. Nonetheless, a huge data set can prove to be a hindrance for good performance using this technique. It is also not easy to interpret the process when compared to that of regression tree.

Asthe Internet-of-Thingspaves a new way of looking at health information, along with advancement in machine learning techniques and algorithms, many systems are being built, so highly advanced, that they could calculate the behaviors of nearly everything, from consumer purchase patterns to the stock market conditions. Hence, such advanced systems in healthcare industry have an enormous opportunity to take advantage of these decision-making abilities [54]. Hence the role played by prescriptive analytics in health-care industry and its associated operations is highly significant. It not only provides the concerned personnel with a wide range of feasible alternatives, it also helps them to look down in time in a particular course of action, assess its opportunities and problems and then choose the best course of action. This enables the executives or users of this technique to be equipped with the right tool to overcome any and all the possible hindrances to a great extent. This translates to monetary benefits and a better utilization of resources.

Exploratory Analytics

It is an approach that analyses data sets to summarize the main characteristics with the help of visual aids. The main objective of exploratory data analytics is to acquire a complete understanding of the data set and highlight its significant features before performing any analysis on them. This process aids to create a hypothesis about the data set itself. This further aids in interpretation of conducted experiments where the analyst or the researcher has no control of over the conditions of objects under investigation. Exploratory data analytic techniques reveal the structure of data set and the association between the different parameters. Visualization of data plays an important role in this approach. It allows the analyst develop correlations between different parameter and form a conclusion regarding the outcome. Often Principal Component Analysis (PCA) technique is employed to visualize the data. This technique allows the data to be represented with a reduction in number of dimensions and without a significant loss of information [55].

TheNational Institute of Standards and Technology (NIST) describe EDAas an approach to data analysis, not a model, that uses these techniques [55]:

- Maximize insights into a dataset.
- Uncover underlying structures.
- Extract important variables.
- Detect outliers and anomalies.
- Test underlying assumptions.
- Develop parsimonious models.
- Determine optimal factor settings.

In the health care industry, exploratory analytic technique can be used to identify the age, gender and genome that is most affected with a certain disease. Box Plots, Scatter plot, Histograms, Heat map and pictograms are the commonly used visual aids to identify trends and pattern within the data set.

To summarize, data-analytics play a huge role in the health care industry. It is used by executives of different domains. This includes top management, doctors, physicians, engineers and accountants. The different analytic techniques discussed above are used in accordance with the need of an institution. Descriptive and diagnostic data analytic techniques are more popular when compared to the rest because of its ease of deployment, readability of insights and usage. That being said, the future trend of data analytics in health care industry lies in proactive approach rendered by predictive and prescriptive data analytics.

CONCLUSION

The focus of this chapter was to provide an overview of health informatics through the perspective of data analytics.In the 21st century, rapid technological advancements are making wave of changes. Medicine certainly is one of the fields which is getting largely benefitted from these wave of changes. While it has become more and more excitable to accrue medical data, large scale efforts are put in to convert this data into sensible knowledge. The three fundamental aspects of healthcare such as care, education and research thrive on computer assisted 3Ds: data collection, discretion in use and decision making.

The first part of the chapter has dealt with the fundamental description of medical data types. On further reading, the readers would explore the common resources of medical data currently available in our society. The chapter also presents an overview of healthcare databases. An entire section is devoted to Electronic Health Records (EHR) that is an abundant source of healthcare data. The structure of EHRs with respect to two most popular standards, openEHR and HL7 has been discussed at length along with a short introduction to the emerging FHIR standard. This chapter presents a discussion on the Indian standards for EHR implementation, which is a new-of-its kind in books of this segment. The application of EHRs in clinical informatics and nursing informatics has been dealt, since these two fields are mutually influential on the implementation and success of EHR systems.

The second part of the chapter provides a comprehensive discussion on the analysis and visualization of healthcare data. A comprehensive review of the stages involved in data processing has been presented to the readers with relevant examples. Apart from data exploration methods, the tools available for performing the data analytics explorations have also been outlined by the authors.An entire section has been devoted to a detailed discussion on the various facets of analytics including, Descriptive Analytics, Diagnostic Analytics, Predictive Analytics and Prescriptive Analytics. Instances of classifiers, clusters and other machine learning methods have been represented adequately such that researchers and students interested in the field of medical informatics can equip themselves with better knowledge.

References

[1] AMIA, "*What is informatics?*" Available at https://www.amia.org/fact-sheets/what-informatics, Accessed March 10, 2020.

[2] Prescient & Strategic Intelligence, "*Digital Health Market Research Report*," https://www.psmarketresearch.com/market-analysis/digital-health-market, Accessed March 10, 2020.

[3] National Library of medicine, "*Health Data Sources*," Available at https://www.nlm.nih.gov/nichsr/stats_tutorial/section3/index.html, March 11, 2020.

[4] *The Complete Medical Record and Electronic Charting*, http://assets.cengage.com/pdf/smp_3510_heller_chapter3.pdf. Accessed March 11, 2020.

[5] *Stanford Medicine Health Trends Report 2020: The Rise of the Data Driven Physician*, Available at https://med.stanford.edu/content/dam/sm/phs/documents/7.%20Joel%20Kallich_%20Optum%20Health%20Care%20Claims%20Data2-1.pdf. Accessed March 11, 2020.

[6] James, R.C., Vignesh, V., Terwilliger, B.A. and Parker, B.C. 2018. "Surgical and Medical Applications of Drones: A Comprehensive Review." *Journal of the Society of Laparoscopic & Robotic Surgeons* 22(3):1-9. doi: 10.4293/JSLS.2018.00018.

[7] Whipple, E.C., McGowan, J.J., Dixon, B.E. and Zafar, A. 2009."The selection of high-impact health informatics literature: a comparison of results between the content expert and the expert searcher." *J Med Libr Assoc*. 97(3):212-218. doi: 10.3163/1536-5050.97.3.010.

[8] Kong, H.J. 2019. "Managing Unstructured Big Data in Healthcare System."*Healthc Inform Res*. 25(1):1-2. doi: 10.4258/hir.2019.25.1.1.

[9] *Database*, https://www.oracle.com/in/database/what-is-database.html, Accessed March 13, 2020.

[10] Lele, R.D. 2005. *Computers in Medicine*.: Tata McGraw Hill.

[11] David, M. G., Lisa, G.S., Robert, J. L., Nazir, L., Judith L. M. and Timothy, S.W. 2018. "Determinants of Health-Related Quality of Life After ICU: Importance of Patient Demographics, Previous Comorbidity, and Severity of Illness." *Critical Care Medicine* 46(4):594-601.

[12] Gian, C. G., Giovanni, P., Antonella, B., Luca, G., Pier, P.B. and Giuseppe, L. 2009. "Development and implementation of an automatic system for verification, validation and delivery of laboratory test results." *Clinical Chemistry and Laboratory Medicine* 47(11):1355-60.

[13] ASPE Inventory of Health Care Information Standards. ASTM E1384-96 Standard Guide for Content and Structure of the Computer-Based Patient Record, https://aspe.hhs.gov/report/inventory-health-care-information-standards/astm-e1384-96-standard-guide-content-and-structure-computer-based-patient-record, Accessed May 13, 2020.

[14] Watzlaf, V.J., Zeng, X., Jarymowycz, C. and Firouzan, P.A. 2004. "Standards for the content of the electronic health record" *Perspect Health Inf Manag*. 1(1).

[15] *The ISO 13606 standard*, http://www.en13606.org/information.html, March 15, 2020.

[16] Electronic Health Record (EHR) Standards For India. 2016. *Standards Set Recommendations* v 2.0, https://www.nrces.in/download/files/pdf/nrces_ehr_stand_india.pdf, Accessed March 15, 2020.

[17] Jeff, H. 2020. "*The future of electronic health records*." Available at https://www.nature.com/articles/d41586-019-02876-y. Accessed March 15, 2020.

[18] Ohno-Machado, L., Kim, J., Gabriel, R.A., Kuo, G.M. andHogarth, M.A. 2018. "Genomics and electronic health record systems." *Human Molecular Genetics* 27: 48–55.

[19] "*What is openEHR?*" https://www.openehr.org/about/what_is_openehr, Accessed March 15, 2020.

[20] Goossen, W. T. 2014. "Detailed clinical models: representing knowledge, data and semantics in healthcare information technology." *Healthc Inform Res.* 20(3):163-172. doi: 10.4258/hir.2014.20.3.163.

[21] https://specifications.openehr.org/releases/RM/latest/ehr.html#_the_ehr_information_model, Accessed March 15, 2020.

[22] About HL7, https://www.hl7.org/about/index.cfm?ref=nav. Accessed March 20, 2020.

[23] White Paper on "*HL7 EHR System Functional Model: A Major Development Towards Consensus on Electronic Health Record System Functionality*," 2004.

[24] *FHIR Foundation Enabling health interoperability through FHIR*, https://fhir.org/, Accessed March 20, 2020.

[25] *EMR-EHR Standards for India*, https://main.mohfw.gov.in/sites/default/files/EMR-EHR_Standards_for_India_as_notified_by_MOHFW_2016_0.pdf,Accessed March 23, 2020.

[26] Plaisant, C., Shneiderman, B. and Mushlin, R. 1998. "An Information Architecture to Support the Visualization of Personal Histories Information." *Management and Processing* 34(5):581-597.

[27] Cui, T., Wei-Qi, W., Harold, R. S., Guergana, S. and Christopher, G. C. 2010. "CNTRO: A Semantic Web Ontology for Temporal Relation Inferencing in Clinical Narratives." *Proc. AMIA Annual Symp.*: 787-791.

[28] Hripcsak, G., Albers, D.J. andPerotte, A. 2011. "Exploiting time in electronic health record correlations." *J Am Med Inform Assoc.* 18: 109–115.

[29] Joshi, R. and Szolovits, P. 2012. "Prognostic physiology: modeling patient severity in intensive care units using radial domain folding." *AMIA Annu Symp Proc.*:1276–1283.

[30] David, G., Jimeng, S., Nan, C. and Shahram, E. 2011. "Visual cluster analysis in support of clinical decision intelligence."*AMIA Annu Symp Proc.*: 481–490.

[31] Jennifer, G. S., Kipp, D., Jordan, D. S., Tessa, F. and Nathaniel, E.L. 2016. "Improving the Efficiency and Ease of Healthcare Analysis Through Use of Data Visualization Dashboards." *Big Data* 4(2): 129-135.

[32] J. An, X. Lu and H. Duan. 2008. "Integrated Visualization of Multi-Modal Electronic Health Record Data." Paper presentedat the *2nd International Conference on Bioinformatics and Biomedical Engineering*, Shanghai: 640-643.

[33] Sittig D. F., Murphy D. R., Smith M. W., Russo E., Wright A. and Singh H. 2015. "Graphical display of diagnostic test results in electronic health records: a comparison of 8 systems." *J Am Med Inform Assoc.* 22(4): 900-904. doi: 10.1093/jamia/ocv013.

[34] Kennell, T., Willig, J.H. and Cimino, J.J. 2017. "Clinical Informatics Researcher's Desiderata for the Data Content of the Next Generation Electronic Health Record." *Appl Clin Inform.* 8(4):1159-1172, doi: 10.4338/ACI-2017-06-R-0101

[35] Thomas, H. P., Sarah, C., Theresa, A.C., Tejal, K.G., Linda, H., Gilad, J.K., John, E.M. 2015. "Report of the AMIA EHR-2020 Task Force on the status and future direction of EHRs." *Journal of the American Medical Informatics Association* 22(5): 1102–1110, https://doi.org/10.1093/ jamia/ocv066.

[36] Kelley, T.F., Brandon, D.H. and Docherty, S.L. 2011. "Electronic nursing documentation as a strategy to improve quality of patient care." *J Nurs Scholarsh.* 43(2):154-62. doi: 10.1111/j.1547-5069. 2011.01397.x.

[37] Susan, M. D. and Anne, M. B. 2013. *Advanced Practice Nursing: Evolving Roles for the Transformation of the Profession*. Jones & Bartlett Publishers.

[38] Benjamin, S., Patrick, J.T., Azra, B. and Parisha, R. 2017 "Deep EHR: A Survey of Recent Advances in Deep Learning Techniques

for Electronic Health Record (EHR) Analysis." *IEEE Journal of Biomedical and Health Informatics*. 22(5): 1589-1604.

[39] Harerimana, G., Kim, J. W., Yoo, H. and Jang, B.2019. "Deep Learning for Electronic Health Records Analytics." *IEEE Access.* 7:101245-101259.

[40] Vuppalapati, C., Ilapakurti, A.and Kedari, S. 2016. "The Role of Big Data in Creating Sense EHR, an Integrated Approach to Create Next Generation Mobile Sensor and Wearable Data Driven Electronic Health Record (EHR)." Paper presented at *IEEE Second International Conference on Big Data Computing Service and Applications (BigDataService),* Oxford: 293-296.

[41] Jensen, P.B., Jensen, L.J. and Brunak, S. 2012. "Mining electronic health records: Towards better research applications and clinical care." *Nat Rev Genet*. 13(6): 395-405. doi: 10.1038/nrg3208.

[42] Lee, C.H. and Yoon, H.J. 2017. "Medical big data: Promise and challenges." *Kidney Res Clin Pract*. 36(1): 3-11. doi: 10.23876/j. krcp.2017.36.1.3.

[43] Gunter, T.D. and Terry, N.P. 2005. "The emergence of national electronic health record architectures in the United States and Australia: models, costs, and questions." *J Med Internet Res*.7(1): e3. doi: 10.2196/jmir.7.1.e3.

[44] Islam, M.S., Hasan, M.M., Wang, X., Germack, H.D. andNoor-E-Alam, M. 2018. "A Systematic Review on Healthcare Analytics: Application and Theoretical Perspective of Data Mining." *Healthcare (Basel)*.6(2):54. doi: 10.3390/healthcare6020054.

[45] Liu, F. T., Ting, K. and Zhou, Z. 2012. "Isolation-Based Anomaly Detection." *ACM Transactions on Knowledge Discovery from Data*. 6: 1-39. 10.1145/2133360.2133363. doi.org/10.1145/2133360. 2133363.

[46] Mangasarian, O. L., Setiono, R. and Wolberg, W.H. 1990."Pattern recognition via linear programming: Theory and application to medical diagnosis." *Large-scale numerical optimization.* Thomas F. Coleman and Yuying Li, editors, SIAM Publications: 22-30.

[47] Raghupathi, W. andRaghupathi, V. 2013. "An Overview of Health Analytics." *J Health Med Informat.* 4: 132. doi: 10.4172/2157-7420. 1000132.

[48] https://healthitanalytics.com/news/healthcare-big-data-analytics-from-description-to- prescription. Date of Access 10-05-2020.

[49] LaValle, S., Lesser, E., Shockley, R., Hopkins, M.S.and Kruschwitz, N. 2013. "Big data, analytics and the path from insights to value." *MIT Sloan Manage Rev*: 21.

[50] https://www.ibm.com/blogs/business-analytics/diagnostic-analytics-101-why-did-it-happen/ Date of Access 10-05-2020.

[51] https://uc-r.github.io.

[52] https://fmcna.com/insights/education/types-of-healthcare-analytics/ Date of Access 28-04-2020.

[53] https://healthtechmagazine.net/article/2019/10/how-predictive-analytics-impacting-patient-care-perfcon. Date of Access 13-04-2020.

[54] https://healthitanalytics.com/news/healthcare-big-data-analytics-from-description-to-prescription.

[55] https://www.mastersindatascience.org/resources/what-is-exploratory-data-analysis/.

In: Computing Paradigms for Smart Healthcare ISBN: 978-1-53618-619-2
Editors: B. Vinoth Kumar et al.

Chapter 2

SMART CONNECTED HOSPITALS – A STEP AHEAD INTO HEALTHCARE 4.0

Bhama Sadhasivam[1], PhD, J. Uma Maheswari[2], PhD and G. R. Karpagam[3], PhD

[1]Department of CA
[2,3]Department of CSE,
PSG College of Technology, Coimbatore, Tamil Nadu, India

ABSTRACT

One of the greatest challenges to be handled in the current environment is the escalating cost of healthcare. As technology meets the needs of humanity, there are changes in the way of working and hence the way of living. Healthcare providers are responsible to enhance the delivery and accessibility of healthcare services, in addition to the basic challenge of care taking of patients. The growth rate of healthcare data is exponential. At times of emergency, patients need to move to different doctors and hospitals. Hence, the patient data is sourced from disparate systems, which may have varied levels of storage, accessibility, transparency and quality. Also, it is often the case that there are discrepancies in the communication of technologies. This triggers the need for connecting hospitals. A 'smart connected environment' includes objects that can store, process and exchange information seamlessly using technologies. Thus, healthcare systems become smart when they link in a smarter way to integrate data at a reasonable cost.

The technology enablers for interconnecting hospitals include,

- Service Oriented Architecture – for efficient communication among hospitals for various processes of the system in terms of healthcare services
- Web Services – for standardizing the interface for data exchange among heterogeneous hospital systems
- Semantics – for increasing the accuracy during discovery of services for the patients
- Facial Recognition – for providing security to the medical record of patients

Keywords: web service, semantics, case-based reasoning, web service discovery, facial recognition, healthcare, smart connectivity

MOTIVATING SCENARIO

The major and critical task of hospital management is the maintenance of health records of patients. Thus, an architecture revealing the necessity of connecting all hospitals together to share the health records is shown in Figure 1:

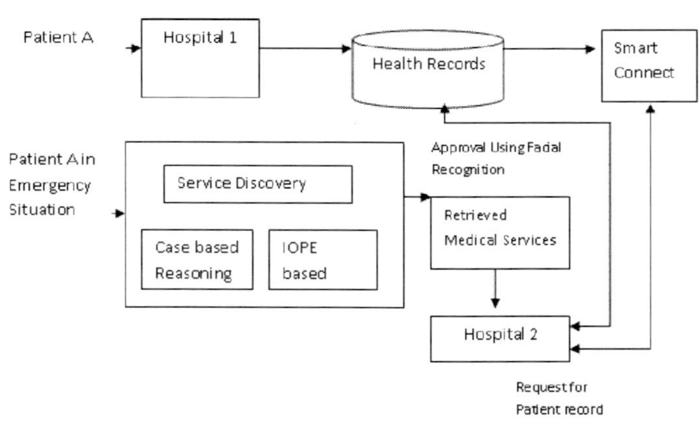

Figure 1. Conceptual Architecture for web services enabled smart connected hospitals.

Consider Patient-A is visiting Hospital-1 regularly and all his health records are stored in Hospital-1's database. In an emergency situation, the patient's relatives are seeking for automated medical services. The medical services are invoked using case-based reasoning and IOPE based Web service discovery. Therefore, it retrieves ambulance service and doctor service. Because of the availability issue, the Patient-A is taken into Hospital-2. There they need previous health records of patients which are available in Hospital-1's database. So here there is a need for a technique which takes care of bringing the required details from Hospital-1 to Hospital-2. In this scenario, Hospital-2 is seeking access to Patient-A's medical records which is stored in Hospital-1 database. The Hospital-1 can give the access rights based on the facial recognition of patients or their relatives. Therefore, the hospitals are connected in a smarter way ensuring secured communication using facial recognition.

Smart Connectivity

'Connectivity' offers a big deal in providing healthcare provision and services. The transformative change due to connectivity extends the ability not just to monitor patients and devices, but also provides opportunity for other technologies such as data analysis and automation. These promise to provide efficiency and flexibility into the provision of healthcare services. With the deployment of technologies of information handling and the need for sharing data among hospitals, smart connectivity aims to provide value-added healthcare services [3].

The adoption of connectivity in the healthcare industry is based on its varied nature of special aspects and concerns. Variations in the healthcare industry may range over the availability of services such as appointment with doctors / specialists, payment modes and so on. Human health is an aspect of paramount importance that necessitates the delivery of affordable healthcare services. The smart healthcare environment is distributed and patient-centric, as shown in the Figure 2:

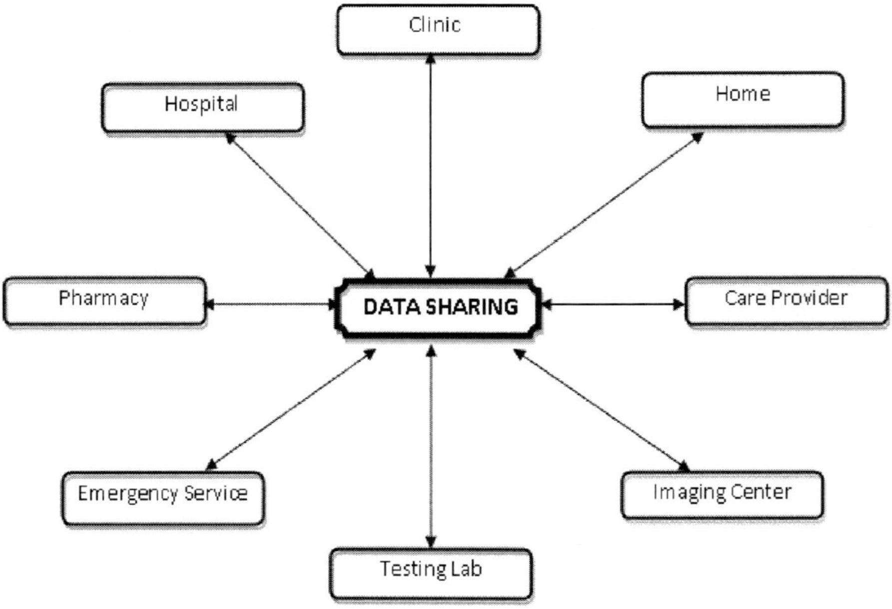

Figure 2. Future of smart healthcare.

In recent years, the notion of smart hospitals is realized by the application of web services [5]. The integration and collaboration of medical facilities is supported by healthcare services. Smart connectivity of hospitals lays an infrastructure for enhancement of processes involved in healthcare management. In addition to embracing the apt technologies, web services provide cost-effective operations for smart connected hospitals.

Smart Healthcare

Smart healthcare is seen as a way of intelligent application of trending technologies which can help the stakeholders connect people, information and healthcare industry [10]. Technological enhancements and digitization do have their impact on the evolution of industries in profound ways and healthcare is no exception. For example, smart hospitals are driven by big data analytics. There is a connectivity identified between the integration of new technologies on the provider's side and the increase in the expectations on the consumer's side. As a result, this has led to the redefinition of healthcare services delivery among smart connected hospitals.

Services for Healthcare

In situations of emergency, including pandemics, natural or man-made disasters or terrorist attacks, healthcare services play a key role. Most disasters have significant impacts on human health, placing additional demands on healthcare services. In order to handle the surge in demand during such an emergency or disaster, the availability of healthcare services is essential. The services related to healthcare may include such facilities that support all aspects of emergency handling such as the preparedness, response and recovery. The provision of emergency healthcare services is a complex task which requires a set of services. As an evolving form of enabling technology, applications based on web services provide an easier way of accessing healthcare services.

Web services enable the sharing of data, which is the basic requirement in the healthcare industry. 942 services have been taken from Web Ontology Language for Services (OWL-S) Test Collection with different domains like medical care, food, travel, communication, weapons and geography which are related to emergency management. This collection is intended to support the evaluation of the performance of case-based reasoning and OWL-S service matchmaking algorithms. Out of 942 services, importance was given to the travel domain because if the patient is in an emergency situation like heart attack then the first service to be invoked is ambulance service from the travel domain and followed by the hospital service which is invoked based on the availability of the doctors. The ambulance and doctor services are invoked based on two methods of service discovery namely, case-based reasoning and Input-Output-Precondition-Effect (IOPE) based. Following sections provide an explanation of the methods.

CASE-BASED REASONING

Reasoning is the process of drawing inferences based on known facts or other intelligible information. A 'case' is a similar set of related facts. Case-Based Reasoning (CBR) is considered as an approach of solving problems based on solutions to other previous similar problems. CBR has evolved as part of the more general field of Artificial Intelligence (AI). The overall objective of AI is to support development of solutions in the form of programs that mimic the general mechanisms of human intelligence. CBR has become popular in the recent years since it provides solutions to problems by considering available solutions to problems of similar nature.

CBR Based Discovery of Services

With the hike in the development of internet technologies, web services have found applications in various domains such as business, healthcare, travel, education and so on. Recent research focuses on adding intelligent techniques so as to enhance discovery, selection and composition of web services.

CBR is an approach in which past experience is used to solve a new problem. The solutions of problems are stored as cases that can be used to address the recent problems. In the context of service discovery, CBR is preferred as one of the approaches because a new request for a service can be handled efficiently. The current request is mapped with similar requests stored in the case base and the relevant services are retrieved.

CBR is a typical model of analogical reasoning in AI. The main focus of CBR is on the semantic similarity in a domain. In general, the major advantages of the CBR approach to problem solving include the following:

- Implementation of CBR system is an easier task of identifying relevant cases

- Reasoning task can start with a partial case base, as its growth is cyclic in nature
- Learning system has case-based nature that leads to makes easier maintenance

CBR – Phases

Following are the four phases in the model of CBR [1] as shown in Figure 3.

- Retrieve older cases where problems have similar features as that of the new problem
- Reuse or Adapt an existing solution suggested by a previous similar case
- Revise or Evaluate the solution and modify it if necessary, to fit the new problem
- Retain or Learn the new solution after its validation or confirmation

Each phase in the lifecycle of CBR follows a certain rule. Initially, CBR receives a new problem to be solved and then finds a solution that exists for a similar problem so as to reuse it. For this, CBR must retrieve similar cases from the case base by determining the similarity of cases in the case base to the new problem. Next, a CBR system should reuse the solution, either with or without revision. Finally, CBR system should retain the new problem and its solution as a case to the case base to increase its knowledge. The case library is assumed to be available, which consists of problems and solutions. The problems are the requested functionalities and the solutions are the corresponding services that satisfy the functionalities [2].

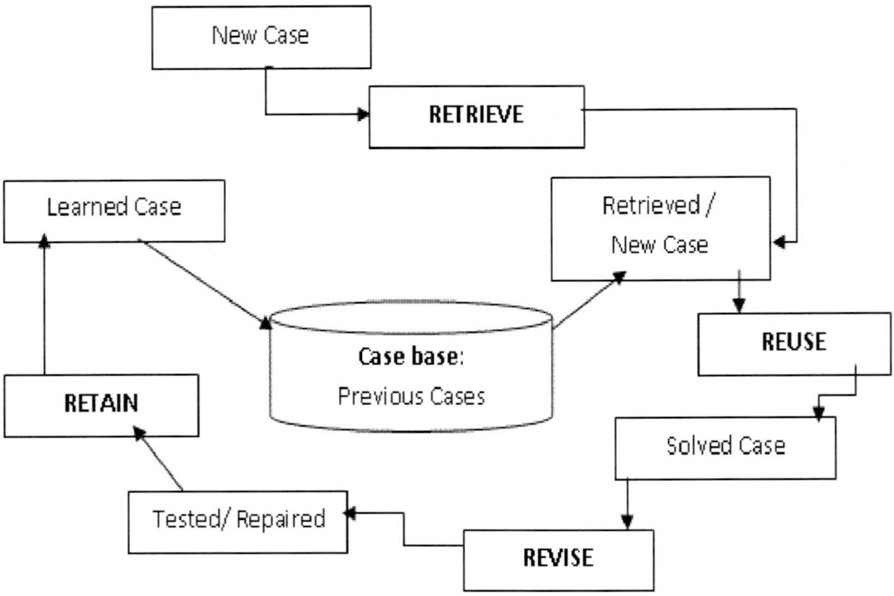

Figure 3. Phases of CBR.

It is assumed that the web services in various domains are registered by the service providers in a common repository. These services need to be classified based on their domain which may be accomplished using a classifier. It applies machine learning algorithms to classify the services in the repository.

Whenever there is a demand from the consumers, their service request is forwarded to the Request Processor. The processor generates a service request vector including the domain of the service which is then passed on to the Reasoner. This is the component that plays the major role in the discovery of desired web services. The case base is a repository of problems and their possible solutions. The Reasoner considers the request as a new case and then does the matchmaking of this request with those available in the case base. If matching cases exist, then they are passed on to the Selector component. It then compares the matched cases with the service parameters by referring to the Classifier output. As a result, it identifies those services that match the consumer's request. After identification of those services that match the request, the list of relevant services is returned to the next phase of the web service called IOPE based web service discovery. For the emergency scenario mentioned above, if the patient is in critical situation, based on the patient's location the ambulance service has been selected by referring to the Classifier output and the set of identified services are passed to the IOPE based service discovery phase.

IOPE Based Service Discovery

The service description consists of the functional description of the web service that includes the inputs that are mandatory for the services to be executed, the information which is generated as the output of the services, pre conditions needed before executing the web services [4] and the final effect after execution of particular service. The requested service parameters like input, output, pre-condition and effect are compared with the functional parameters of the service which are stored in the repository by the service providers using Word Net. Instead of matching the exact words in the request and stored service, the synonyms [6] of the word are used for comparison in order to increase the accuracy of matching. The purpose of Word Net is as follows.

Word Net

WordNet is a database which groups English words into sets of synonyms called synsets. It also gives the relations among these synonym sets. WordNet [7] can be inferred and used as a lexical ontology. The hypernym/hyponym relationships among the synsets can be interpreted as specialization relations.

Words and Synsets

A word is a collection of senses. Each sense is captured as a set of word-senses that are synonymous, or a synset. So, a word is a set of synsets. To retrieve a word from WordNet, use synsets (<word>). For example, the following returns a list of synsets, each of which captures a sense associated with the word 'dog':

```
wn.synsets('dog')
[Synset('dog.n.01'), Synset('frump.n.01'), Synset('dog.n.03'),
Synset('cad.n.01'), Synset('frank.n.02'), Synset('paw1.n.01'),
Synset('andiron.n.01'), Synset('chase.v.01')]
```

where wn is a wordnet object. Each synset is labelled with a 3-part name of the form <word>.<pos>.<number>, where <word> is the word, <pos> is the part-of-speech of the word, <number> is the index of the sense. For example, 'dog.n.01' means the first meaning of 'dog' used as a noun.

Using the above function, the synsets for the user input, output, pre-condition and effect of the needed services are found and those words are matched with the input, output, pre-condition and effect parameters of the stored services in the repository. If there is a match, then the score is assigned as 1. The procedure is repeated for all 4 functional parameters. Then the overall score is calculated and the services are ranked.

Figure 4 represents the process of IOPE based service discovery. For the scenario where the patient is in emergency situation and he needs ambulance service, first the case-based reasoning method was invoked. Based on the distance or the location of the patient, the similar cases have been identified using classification and the resultant services (constituting the set of similar services where the distance from the patient location to the hospital was minimum) are returned to IOPE based service discovery [8]. In this phase, the parameters such as input, output, pre-condition and effect for the requested services are matched with the synonyms of the stored services. If there is exact word match or synonym match, then the score is assigned as 1 for input parameter. Same procedure is repeated for all parameters and all synonyms. Based on the added score of all four parameters, the aggregated score is calculated and the services are ranked accordingly in descending order. The ambulance service with the highest score is invoked and the patient is transferred to the hospital using the invoked ambulance service. The doctor in that hospital wishes to refer to the previous medical records of the patient which are stored in another hospital's database. Then the request is sent to the old hospital by the doctor from the new hospital. The old hospital requests for face authorization of the patient or their relatives to reveal the particular patient's medical records. If the face of the patient or relative matches with the faces which are stored in the old hospital database for the corresponding patient, then immediately the old hospital transfers the medical records to the new hospital. The process of facial recognition is as follows.

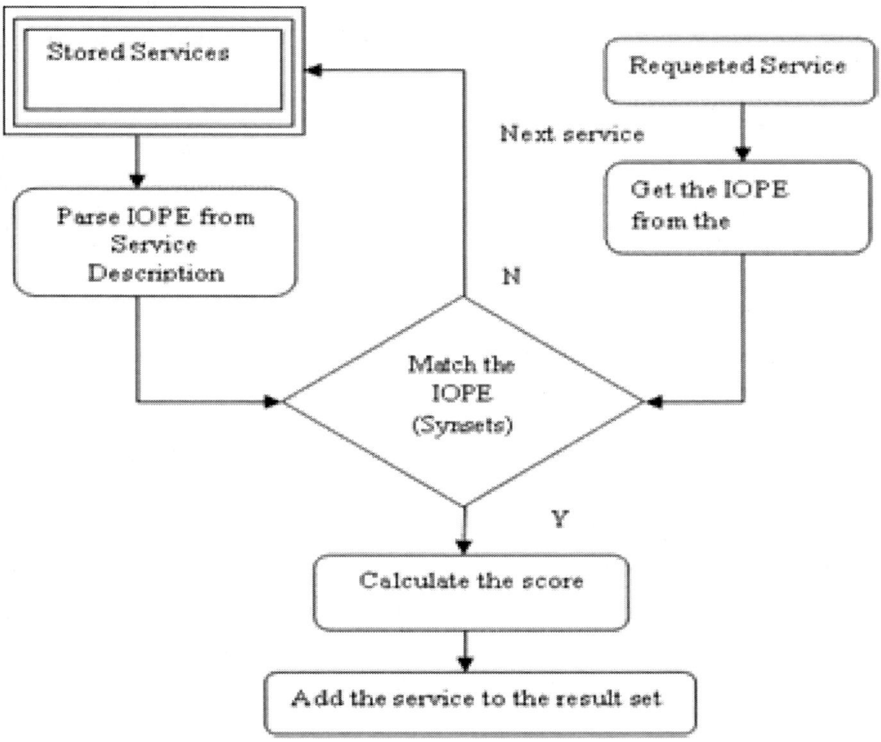

Figure 4. IOPE based service discovery.

FACIAL RECOGNITION

With the rapid development of AI in recent years, facial recognition gains increased attention. Facial recognition is contactless, cost effective, highly concurrent and user friendly which are advantageous when compared with the traditional fingerprint recognition and iris recognition. It is preferred to be used in government, public facilities such as medical care, e-commerce, education, insurance, security, retailing and many other fields.

Facial recognition requires capturing face image and comparison with the stored images in the database. Initially, the system should be trained with known images, and then the images are classified with known classes which are stored in the database. When a test image is given to the system, it is classified and compared with stored images in the database.

Automatic facial recognition involves face detection, feature extraction and face recognition. The Eigen face method [9] is based on the reduction of face-dimensional space using Principal Component Analysis (PCA) for facial features.

The general steps for performing the Eigen faces include,

(i) Input a set of images

(ii) Compute covariance matrix of input images

(iii) Extract Eigen faces from the image data using PCA

(iv) Represent each image as a vector of weights

(v) Calculate the weight of the unknown image is and then compare to the weights of those images already in the database. If the input image weight is over a given threshold it is considered to be unknown. The identification of the input image is done by finding the image in the database which has the closest weight of the input image, which is the one that belongs to that particular person. If there is a match, the doctor from the new hospital is allowed to access the medical records of the patient which are stored in the old hospital's database.

Conclusion

This chapter provides an insight into smart connectivity of hospitals using appropriate technologies such as case-based reasoning, IOPE based service discovery and facial recognition. It also addresses the issues of healthcare providers who are responsible to enhance the delivery and accessibility of healthcare services, in addition to the basic challenge of care taking of patients. The Case-based and IOPE based service discovery methods ensure the accuracy and relevancy of services which are retrieved and invoked for patients. Facial recognition system guarantees the security of patients' healthcare information. The system can be further extended by combining IoT and blockchain based technologies to give more smartness to healthcare systems.

References

[1] Aamodt, A. E. Plaza, 1994, "Case-Based Reasoning: Foundational Issues, Methodological Variations, and System Approaches", *AI Communications*. IOS Press, Vol. 7: 1, pp. 39-59.

[2] De Renzis, Alan, Martin Garriga, Andres Flores, Alejandra Cechich, 2016, "Case-based Reasoning for Web Service Discovery and Selection", *Electronic Notes in Theoretical Computer Science*, 321, pp. 89–112.

[3] Bokolo, Anthony Jnr., 2020, "A Case-Based Reasoning Recommender System for Sustainable Smart City Development", *AI & Society*.

[4] Bettina, F. and Thomas, L. 2010, "Semantic search on the Web, Semantic Web — Interoperability, Usability, Applicability", *IOS Press*, pp. 1-7.

[5] Douglas, K and David D, 2013, "Web Services, Service-Oriented Architectures, and Cloud Computing: The Savvy Manager 's Guide", *Elsevier*.

[6] Grigoris, A, and Frank V, 2004, "A Semantic Web Primer", *The MIT Press*, Cambridge.

[7] Princeton University, 2010, "*About WordNet*", Available from: http://wordnet.princeton.edu.

[8] Uma, J. Maheswari and GR Karpagam, 2015, "Cloud Based Comprehensive Architecture (CBCA) for QoS Aware Semantic Web Service Discovery in Emergency Management System." *International Journal of Applied Engineering Research,* Vol. 10: 23, pp. 43763-43771.

[9] Kamencay, Patrik, Miroslav Benco, Tomas Mizdos, Roman Radil, 2017, "A New Method for Face Recognition Using Convolutional Neural Network", *Digital Image Processing and Computer Graphics*, doi: 10.15598/aeee. v15i4.2389.

[10] Tian, Shuo, Wenbo Yang, Jehane Michael Le Grange, Peng Wang, Wei Huang, Hewed Ye, 2019, "Smart healthcare: making medical care more intelligent", *Global Health Journal*, Vol. 3: 3, pp. 62-65.

In: Computing Paradigms for Smart Healthcare ISBN: 978-1-53618-619-2
Editors: B. Vinoth Kumar et al.

Chapter 3

An Intelligent Healthcare System for Automatic Diagnosis of Diseases Based on Deep Learning with IoT Enabled Cloud Computing Framework

S. K. Somasundaram*[*]*, PhD

Department of Information Technology, PSG College of Technology, Coimbatore, Tamil Nadu, India

Abstract

The utilization of Intelligent Healthcare frameworks is ubiquitous due to the widespread of Internet of Things (IoT) and fast progressions in Information Technology. As a multifaceted, all day facility, healthcare entails proficient and solid sequel on day by day tasks, administration and assets. Cloud and edge-based computing are basic for intelligent and proficient medicinal services frameworks in shrewd urban areas. The IoT

* Corresponding Author's Email: sks.it@psgtech.ac.in.

framework gathers patient status such as temperature, pressure, body sugar level, pulse rate and so forth from their associated clinical gadgets. The data acquired from the gadgets are pre-processed and transferred to a centralized or decentralized network. Deep learning-built representations with extremely high precision necessitate exceedingly huge computing resources for both training and testing. The proposed work permitted multifaceted deep learning networks to be entrenched in cloud paradigms using innovative communication and typical dissemination methods like collaborating in which high precision to be accomplished with remarkably low latencies. The real-time patient data is authenticated by investigating the trained neural networks on standard datasets and installing an operational structure that affords prediction outcomes in real-time. A cloud framework is used to corroborate the system and to test the effectiveness of suggested system in terms of training precision, testing precision, latency time, intercession time, power consumption characteristics and network bandwidth.

Keywords: intelligent healthcare system, deep learning, IoT, cloud computing framework, clinical gadgets

INTRODUCTION

Internet of Things (IoT) is an emerging system that synchronizes equipment, acquiring gadgets, sensory devices, programming projects, and creatures or individuals over a system endowing them to cooperate, convey, collect and transfer information. There is a rambling number of clients, administrations and uses related with IoT across various orders [1, 2]. IoT was developed from Radio Frequency Identification (RFID) [3] and Wireless Sensor Network (WSN) innovations [4, 5, 6, 7, 8, 9] to further developed coordination with distributed computing, Internet administrations, digital frameworks and interconnectivity among equipment and programming gadgets [3]. A commonplace IoT framework comprises of sensors, correspondence boundaries, propelled calculations, and cloud border. Sensors and routers were utilized to gather information from various gadgets. RFID innovation and WSN advances give the methods for correspondences and system framework. A considerable number of client server sales can be exchanged between mobiles and organizations in the cloud and web, as such allowing customers to pick up induction to different sorts of organizations at the same time [1, 2, 10, 11].

There are distinctive significant kinds of IoT benefits as follows [1, 10, 12, 13, 14, 15]. To begin with, sagacious wearable contraptions can be used for patients who need to assemble data about their prosperity status, for instance, heartbeat, body temperature level and glucose level through sensors on the wearable enhancements, which are sent to mobile devices. The patients' health status can be observed simultaneously. Next, home automation can be triggered by IoT, where sensing devices can distinguish the adjustments in temperature, cooling frameworks can be checked. Home surveillance cameras can catch any gate crashers and send the admonitions to the mortgage holders by portable applications. Subsequently, traffic and conveyance frameworks can be observed by IoT to accomplish smart urban areas. Information can be gathered and investigated to comprehend the updates in rush hour gridlock systems and transportation frameworks. Forward, gracefully chain framework can work with IoT in which all the transmissions were logged and monitored continuously. At the point when merchandise have been transported to the goal, the conveyance records can be stayed up with the latest. Then, the e-banking can operate with dependable outsider instalment frameworks on the cell phones. These utilization instances of IoT can be recorded to a conventional model where this nonexclusive model is to give a simpler mix various administration consistently, running from sensors to arrange framework, and from APIs to enormous information handling, lastly from investigation to prescient demonstrating [1, 16, 17]. This methodology guarantees that clients can have simpler access to administrations, can screen the advancement of the administration conveyance, and can analyze costs and evaluations offered by specialist co-ops. Also, specialist organizations can be increasingly presented to supplementary clients, chequered their commercial execution and check the trend pattern among all the more effectively [10, 16, 17]. Models incorporate Gpay, Phonepe, Amazon pay, Pay Pal, and Paytm that clients can buy and wage in practically no time. Clients can have more assortments of alternatives for their buy and have an increasingly helpful approach to finish their exchanges all the more effectively without a need to go the merchant straightforwardly.

Smart health protection is one of the significant parts of intelligent urban communities. The extent of shrewd health protection rises up out of the need to improve the administration of human services division, better use its assets, and diminish its expense while keeping up or in any event, upgrading its eminence level. Assets in the human services segment can comprehensively be grouped to useable assets and non-useable assets. Useable assets incorporate those assets that they rot and lapse by stage like every single clinical guide and apparatuses. Non-consumable assets, then again, are those assets that do not terminate by interval. Amongst the non-useable assets are the HR, for example, doctors, medical caretakers, enlisted attendants and all the human capital engaged with the procedure of medicinal services. The human capital of the healthcare area is an over the top expensive asset and using this asset in a productive manner was a stride moving forward to the total intelligent medicinal services framework.

Throughout the most recent span, the incredible augmentation in grown-ups experiencing incessant sicknesses drastically expanded the need to discover imaginative ways to deal with handle the procedure of human services in a manner to be intelligent as for administration effectiveness and cost [18]. The idea of the healthcare division requires a dependable and proficient approach to manage the gigantic measure of information constantly. On account of cloud and edge processing, planning and creating intelligent healthcare is presently conceivable meanwhile it has been demonstrated that cloud is additional add-on than conventional servers. Moreover, the protection of patients was made possible by distributed computing benefactors [19]. The chances and difficulties of embracing new advances are assessed in [20], and advantages of relocation from customary human services focal frameworks into circulated cloud-Fog based healthcare frameworks, and the comparing requirement for asset designation, bearing and technique, are additionally talked about. Besides, with the help of versatile distributed computing, remote body territory systems can be upgraded for arrangement of human services applications [21]. Cloud and edge registering give a protected, safe, stage for intelligent human services. In a well ahead investigation, Tuan et al. [22] featured and showed the significance of the Internet of Things (IoT) and cloud computing to give superior dependable well-being administrations.

Smart health protection examination can comprehensively be ordered into two principle classifications: patient correlated class and procedure allied classification. Understanding related classification incorporates yet is not constrained to look into that objectives wearable gadgets for gathering information about patients to be accounted for to clinical organizations. Instances of investigation in this classification is the effort of Esposito et al. [23]. In their suggested work, they build up a shrewd portable self-designing engineering that permits swift close to home well-being checking utilizing the ongoing advancements in sensors and versatile implanted gadgets. The creators in [24] examine the significance of wearable gadgets and presentations to gather information about patients' conditions which is obviously bolstered by edge, distributed computing and IoT [25]. Likewise, Shah et al. demonstrate the significance of IoT and intelligent gadgets in enlightening healthcare administrations [26]. Besides, another model in their exploration under this class is represented by Sodhro et al. They build up a solitary electronic based remote observing framework to gather continuous information and screen human statuses [27].

The next classification is the procedure related investigation. In this classification, investigate is worried about the improvement of arrangements to guarantee many angles in the medicinal services area. Among those viewpoints are asset use, asset booking, nature of administration and numerous different angles identified with process definition and the executives. In their effort, they predict the significance of IoT in telemedicine and recommend a structural model for an IoT-based well-being remedies. The model encourages patients to appropriately follow specialists' suggestions [28]. Modern procedures vie for assets [29] while attempting to keep up a necessary hearty quality degree of offered types of assistance [30]. Human services frameworks are vibrant and assorted frameworks that have unusual conduct and that is the reason healthcare frameworks need to deal with their assets and administrations effectively. As referenced before, we characterize assets in two principle classifications: useable and non-useable. Useable assets are those that terminate through routine, including medicines, bedsteads, sheets, chairs and whatever other things that have an expiry date and cannot be public, while non-useable assets, for example, human work, and do not lapse. This examination centers around the procedure level and especially on demonstrating the procedure of asset task in a catastrophe office. To accomplish, we signify Petri nets as a system to demonstrate our procedures and convention.

Controlling the stream procedure in a catastrophe is not unimportant since the framework dynamic conduct is perplexing. A control stream procedure to keep up synchronization among exercises utilizing Petri nets is presented and applied their proposed system on human services segment [31]. Petri nets are graphically spoken to numerical structures to speak to frameworks that are simultaneous.

Emergency action Departments (EaD) are demonstrated utilizing Petri nets. One of the features in EaD is the Length of Remain (LoR), which brings the normal holding up time of patients up, when it rises. This reasons stuffing, which, thus, prompts understanding disappointment [31]. Expanding the limit of EDs and including additional assets is a potential arrangement, however these alternatives are not constantly accessible because of spending requirements and the significant expenses of giving additional offices [32]. This rouses the creators of this chapter to focus on the issue of asset task and procedure displaying and the board of an EaD utilizing Petri nets. In their procedure, additional Petri net subordinate Resource Preservation Net (RPN) is proposed. The examination utilizes re-enactment to demonstrate the possibility of the proposed system to decrease holding up period and patient's LoR throughout stopovers to the EaD with an assistance of cloud innovation. The procedure eases stuffing and lessens the misuse of assets [33].

Inside and outside EaD forms are mimicked, including enlistment, assessment, ophthalmology and charging. The EaD comprises of binary structures associated by a dissident passage, and each structure has a different predicament room. The EaD assists in extra patients yearly, and is available throughout the day. The RPN without anyone else is a scientific built system that we practice to demonstrate the issue of non-useable asset task. The RPN is intended to show the issue of non-useable assets and dole out them on requirement basis. The fundamental commitment of this subordinate of Petri net is to guarantee that non-useable assets are constantly safeguarded, and the framework is free from any danger. The adequacy of RPN is upheld with a couple of characterized Hypotheses. The sufficiency of RPN is not just subject to the arrangement of Petri net and its principal checking yet additionally on the abilities required by the endeavor task and the asset capacities accessible.

In the event that the originator follows the requirements characterized by the statements proposed, the resulting framework is destined to be free from any potential harm. The RPN is coordinated with edge registering where each asset has their individual intelligent gadget that speaks with the cloud regarding that asset status to educate the cloud. At the point when asset is relegated, the cloud guides the task solicitation to the nodes and, when the asset gets sluggish, the node advises the cloud for accompanying task. They incorporate a procedure displaying approach where RPN with the node registering structure for enhanced execution and sophisticated dependability.

Cloud processing standards have risen as a spine of present-day thrift and use internet to give on-request administrations to clients [34]. Both of these spaces have caught noteworthy consideration of enterprises and the scholarly world. But distributed computing is certifiably not a decent alternative for applications requiring continuous reaction due to its high time delay. Innovative advancements like Internet of Things (IoT), Cloud computing, and Big Data have picked up significance because of their strength and capacity to give assorted reaction qualities dependent on track application [36]. These rising advances give stockpiling, calculation, and correspondence to edge gadgets, which encourage and improve versatility, protection, security, low potential, and system data transfer capacity with the goal that Fog registering can splendidly coordinate inactivity delicate or constant applications. Presently, distributed computing structures likewise stretch out help to rising application ideal models, for example,

IoT, Big Data, and cloud processing through assistance and foundation [37, 38]. Cloud computing utilizes switches, process nodes and entryways to offer types of assistance with least conceivable vitality utilization, arrange inertness and reaction interval.

Mutlag et al. [37] investigated the difficulties in health-related submissions and recognized that dormancy and reaction interval are the best significant and hard to enhance Quality of Service (QoS) attributes continuously. Medicinal services are one among the unmistakable presentation zones that involves precise and constant outcomes, which prompts an optimistic advancement. With Fog registering, we carry the assets earlier to the clients along these lines diminishing the idleness and accordingly expanding the security measure. Getting faster outcomes suggests quick activities for basic heart patients. In any case, quicker conveyance of results is not sufficient similarly as with such fragile information we cannot bargain with the precision of the outcome. One approach to get high correctness is by utilizing best in class investigation virtual products commonly that utilize deep learning and its variations prepared on an enormous data source. In ongoing years, deep learning [38] has developed exponentially in the fields going from PC vision [39] to discourse acknowledgment, however has all the more as of late been demonstrated helpful in regular linguistic handling, arrangement forecast, and blended methodology information settings. In addition, deep learning [40] is utilized to outdo numerous classifiers. The storing classifier is one among the outfit strategies where the evaluator hysterics prepares the base classifier on irregular subclasses of information and afterward totals their discrete forecasts either by casting a ballot or by median to get the last expectation. Such evaluators aids in diminishing the change when contrasted with a solitary evaluator by bringing irregularity into the conveyance system of the data source.

Added progression of deep learning is to anticipate and cluster medicinal services information with amazingly high precision [38]. In any case, ongoing models of deep learning for medicinal services presentations are exceptionally sophisticated and entail enormous amount of processing assets for both preparing and forecast [41]. It likewise requires some investment to prepare these complex neural systems and investigate information utilizing it. The more advanced system has higher exactness and forecast time [42] which has been a significant issue for medicinal services and comparative applications of IoTs to acquire brings about ongoing. As calculation on the Edge has the incredible bit of leeway of diminishing reaction time, this provides another guidance of investigation of incorporating multifaceted gathering models of deep learning with Edge Computing to some extent that can get high exactness from constant. The noticeable points of this effort are to overcome this issue and give a processing stage that not just gives less inertness outcomes by utilizing edge assets yet in addition can utilize deep learning-based systems to give exceptionally precise outcomes. There has been some effort to transfer estimation to the devices, closer to the patient to decrease result conveyance time. A portion of these efforts despite everything rely upon re-enactments [42] and have not given convey capable system. This work additionally intends to fill this vacuum in healthcare area.

The remaining of chapter is structured as follows. *Section 2 re*presents existing works on healthcare systems. The proposed model is presented in *Section 3. Section 4* deliberates the experimental setup and represented the results of performance evaluation. *Section 5* discusses conclusions with future work proposed.

RELATED WORKS

Exposures of IoT in Healthcare

Healthcare at the Present Time

An enormous bit of the world's regions is standing up to a noteworthy test to manage the rapidly growing developing masses, individuals with perpetual conditions, adolescent mortality, visit changes of affliction pandemics, and severe day to day environments with poor mental sufficiency, nonattendance of drinking water resources and rising tainting.

Regardless of the way that, the world's enthusiasm for clinical organizations has climbed starting late, we notwithstanding everything live in the standard model of crisis facility driven thought, in which occupants visit pros when they fall cleared out. To manage their consistent affliction, patients make visit to emergency centers or offices for the experts to make reference to target realities that join watching infirmity development and besides to choose clinical decisions that lead to treatment changes. When in doubt, emergency centers use a sickness and specialist centered model that is dynamically responsive and do exclude patients as a working bit of the clinical method.

The following are the possibilities of the difficulties and boundaries considered by clinic driven clinical perform:

- Restricted time and premeditated:
  Growing open with maladies and impairments limits the specialists to look each patient with a value time. In view of the short screening time, specialists do not have the patient's step by step plan, such as, physical activity, rest, diet, and open movement, these qualities are likewise noteworthy in the time taken for examination, analysis and action.
- Obedience observing:
  Specialists were not well equipped to analyze their patients that they were clinging to suggested treatment that may consolidate drugs, rebuilding exercises, and some protective events, for instance, avoiding some eating routine. It is typical that the nonattendance of obedience raises the possibilities of hospitalization [45] and from this time forward, forms the fiscal load to the patients and their families.
- Inhabitants Age:
  Worldwide, the mass of individual with age group more than 60 years (Aged people) is required to progress enormously in excess of 2 billion of every 2050 [46]. In this manner, aged people will search for additional offices and possessions for clinical deliberation.

- Development in Health care:
  By 2030, WHO predicts that 80% of total world population will live in cities and towns [47]. It suggests large metropolitan societies will appeal extra healthcare foundation to aid mounting inhabitants. Additionally, huge metropolitan societies may turn into a focal point of pandemic cataclysms of contagious diseases that may blowout commendably across abundant populaces.
- Healthcare employees Scarcity:
  As the demand for healthcare organizations increases, it likewise grows the demand for health-care workers including clinicians, medical experts, dentists, nurses, support associates, capable gatekeepers, and research office staff who could redesign the human administrations condition in cities, towns and provincial locales. One of the choices as opposed to this test is to fabricate the establishment of tele-medicine.
- Increasing therapeutic rate:
  Undoubtedly the greatest factor in the preventive medicine nowadays is increasing price tag for the human services. For instance, in USA, the expenditure for caring diabetes patients is soaring and is expected to raise to a considerable percentage in the years to come. [48].

IoT-Driven Medical management: Changeover to Patient-Centric

In 1988, the Picker Institute created Patient Centered Care (PCC) for medical services which later become one of the rising models for medicinal services today. The PCC model spotlights on the patients and their distinct human service requirements. In 2001 milestone analysis [49] from Institute of Medicine additionally characterized the PCC as "*Health-care that forms an organization including clinicians, medical experts, dentists, nurses, patients, and their families.*"

PCC demands that patients be collaborators in their personal consideration. Notwithstanding various exercises that give supportive confirmation of PCC and its accomplishment in humbler to-medium scales, we were off by far to recognizing PCC from a certified viewpoint since clinic centered model occurs composed and conflicts with PCC. Nonetheless, fortunately PCC is not intended to kill emergency clinics and facilities. Rather PCC practice it in the mutual template for tenacious consideration. In PCC, to honestly incorporate patients with emergency clinics or centers, there is an essential to practice the amazing biological system of IoT. As depicted before, IoT is an assembly of actuators, sensors, media transmission, distributed computing, Internet communication to give objective arranged administrations. Despite the fact that IoT is a change in outlook system, essentially it is characterized by a working application. Consequently, IoT might be customized to investigate and reduce the difficulties of medicinal services.

Figure 3 shows the characterization of healthcare space, partitioning into tri-zones: 1) huge medicinal services associations, for example, emergency clinics, 2) little facilities and apothecaries, and 3) non-clinical arenas such as houses of the patients, networks, treatment centers, and provincial territories with no clinical help. To imagine IoT's job in human services industry, it is imperative to distinguish the tasks of every one of its territories. When IoT will make a particular activity cost-effective, dependable and auspicious, it will in the long run advance to affect different tasks, structuring a self-reasonable environment for the present battling clinical consideration. In the accompanying, we will take a voyage through possibilities zones where IoT advancements could assume an influential job:

- *Clinics*: For essential consideration, patients will to their general known doctors (family doctors) who currently might exploit IoT from various perspectives. For instance, the experts could essentially get to the patient's health parameters before their visit to the centers. Center gatherings and clinical gatherings to set arrangements for online appointments. IoT will give a minimal effort answer for centers to have an associated checking for its patients so the doctor might invest their greatest knowledge they gained with their patients. Doctors might recommend reasonable

IoT gadgets for self-testing their patients in their respective home which progress towards PCC.

- *Sickbays*: Sickbays are expanding with assets to concede, examine, work or screen expanding quantity of patients. To perform their tasks easily, they continually depend on cutting edge innovations. For instance, intelligent ambulances might accomplish on-armada finding to such an extent that clinicians can prepare few potential ground plans beforehand the appearance of patient, with the incorporation of IoT. Intelligent ambulances might require a lot of dependable clinical devices for conclusion, a safe correspondence connect with medical clinic, and smart work process the executives' instruments for emergency clinic arrangements that may incorporate a working room, where a specialist thinks about the state of the patient well ahead of time. Medical procedures could turn out to be progressively relevant and productive with IoT when the data trade among specialists, clinical staff, and clinical gadgets in working room organize with each other easily. Correspondingly, one can imagine the job of IoT in different divisions of the clinic, for example, emergency unit), (essential consideration unit, and particular units.
- *Everywhere (Without proper clinical Backgrounds):* Bunches of considerations nowadays is about the usage of IoT in online or tele-health care, where the patients are relied upon to increase the following enormous advantages:
    - *Portable hospitals:* There is an expanding enthusiasm for portable well-being centers over the globe. For instance, in African nations, portable centers are proven to offer a minimal effort, top notch care for helpless populaces in remote zones where residents have no entrance to essential clinical offices [50]. Be that as it may, portable centers are vehicles with constrained clinical offices. IoT could have a major effect in improving the framework of the portable facilities that could join forces with huge medical clinics to remotely convey for

determination and choice help. Along these lines, versatile facilities could scale up their abilities for care.

- *Robustness:* The old saying "addressing the issue beforehand is better than addressing any aftermath later" is so obvious and fits properly with the present condition of healthcare. Total populace is turning out to be increasingly mindful that it is smarter to follow anticipatory activities and be positive about individual's well-being than living with drugs, torment, and enduring after that in life. Worldwide residents are marching forward to most of the trend setting innovations, for example, wearable identifiers, sports watches, and self-analyzing clinical gadgets that are likewise arranged as IoT gadgets since they give associated, constant observing of individual's well-being and health. IoT might help fabricate an affordable plan for protection inclusion to control the human services cost dependent on well-being rewards, produced from the well-being following. This could be one of numerous approaches to elevate worldwide populaces to be accomplices of medicinal services framework, setting up a progressively productive patient-focused consideration.
- *Telemedicine*: No ifs, ands or buts, the telemedicine is one of the as a matter of first importance partners of IoT today. As per an ongoing report [51], the worldwide market for telemedicine is expected to develop by 18.8% by the year 2021 with a worth more than $66 million. IoT consumes a great deal to suggest in this field on the grounds that a huge part of total populace owns phones and cell phones, which are not negligible specialized gadgets, yet in addition utilized for interfacing with different sensors. On account of clinical consideration, cell phones are assuming an indispensable job by empowering patients to perform individual examination of their personal well-being. The individual test information develops significant indicators of well-being and ailments. In addition, doctors and clinical staff have approaches to see their

patients with remotely coordinating. IoT could additionally enlarge telemedicine by systems administration sensors to encourage tele-screening. Along these lines, the medical clinics despite everything could get by with fewer quantities of health-care labors by expanding the simulated virtual consideration administrations.

- *Insolent family unit:* Meanwhile the tele-medicine administrations might lessen the quantity of appointments to emergency clinics and centers, particularly for aged patients with interminable circumstances or handicaps, it gets fundamental to set up a specialized foundation in their places. Thus, there should be shrewd places in their houses, offering unpretentious help frameworks to empower residents to encounter freedom, action, personal satisfaction or prosperity. In Europe, Ambient Assisted Living (fruitful shrewd homes system) is hypothesized as encompassing knowledge planned for improving individuals' capacities utilizing delicate, versatile, and responsive computerized conditions [52, 53, 54]. As a rule, IoT has infiltrated the market of home mechanization to give intelligent abilities to inhabitants to control the apparatuses utilizing cell phones and remote controls [55]. Besides, IoT could be redone to satisfy explicit medicinal services needs of older people. Intelligent toilets could accomplish urine examination on standard reason for precautionary and essential consideration. Intelligent homes might change illuminations and echoes to stay away from tactile over-burdens for people with chemical imbalance who at that point might live healthier life.
- *Intelligent metropolises and coupled societies:* The fast relocation of monstrous populace to urban locales has raised the requests and difficulties on the planet's biggest urban communities [47]. Henceforth, rising endeavors are made over the globe to construct shrewd urban communities [56, 57] and associated networks [58] by coordinating and interfacing

different foundations to improve bearableness, supportability, moderateness, and effectiveness. IoT structures are utilized and redone for intelligent urban areas to give the correct data at the perfect spot and at the ideal time to settle on a correct choice to help residents all the more rapidly [59, 60]. As the healthcare framework is a vital piece of urban communities and urban conditions, it has been woven naturally into the textures of smart urban communities and networks in various manners. For instance, urban communities have condition sensors disseminated in their foundation, spilling the sensor information to a unified area such as cloud servers which might now be used by health-care structure. The entrance to the health sensors might mark residents mindful of the circumstances, for example, toxins, dust, temperature, dampness, and water tainting. IoT might convey this data continuously to stay away from and forestall medical problems ahead of time. For example, asthma patients might be made aware of abstain from being in the arenas with high elements (dust/residue) [61]. With a similar methodology, it is conceivable to decrease the force of malignant growth in lungs of the individuals [62]. One another case of how an IoT-driven intelligent urban area might brand the medicinal services progressively proficient is the intermingling of shrewd traffic indicators and emergency vehicle steering to spare survives with the participation of conveyance grounds [63].

In the medicinal services setting, structuring a productive IoT-based framework is a difficult errand because of the accompanying principle issues. To start with, the picked sensor organizing innovation must be asset productive and altered for e-Health presentations. Clinical sensor devices, particularly with the ones that were embedded, have a lot of less organizing power, memory capacity, communication speed, and vitality flexibly than the other sensors in sensor systems area. Next, not at all like basic sensor systems where interim based information transmission is utilized (e.g., temperature and dampness observing), e-health presentations regularly need to oversee overflowing based transmissions where real-time prerequisites should be thought of. Thusly an impressive vitality is dispersed during the transmission procedure. For example, ECG signal transmission requires 4kbps data transfer capacity per channel. Subsequently, in multi-tolerant applications, for example, in intelligent clinics, equipment stages with a more preparing force and equal handling highlights (e.g., multi-center processors) are required in the entryway because of simultaneous nature of the outstanding tasks at hand. Be that as it may, as we talk about in this area, the current broadly useful gateways are not intended for such situations. Succeeding, dependability in e-health presentation is of most extreme significance and even tiny framework inaccessibility regularly cannot go on without serious consequences. Accordingly, as we talk about in the accompanying, the restricted assets of clinical sensor nodes render the utilization of universally useful doors wasteful by and large as for adjournment, vitality, and dependability.

Utilizing a three-level engineering, with shifting computational limit, for IoT presentations is normal in both the manufacturing units and examination. The convergence point of the greater portions of the related works is the gateway utilized in the centre level of the IoT engineering. One of many such endeavors is introduced in [64, 65], which suggests passages to straightforwardly associate sensor systems with various conventions, for example, ZigBee, Wi-Fi, Bluetooth, WiMAX, and Ethernet to the Internet. Be that as it may, these entryways consume self-conscious facility as it might not be modified for numerous presentations. In a different cataloguing of allied work, a passage SwissGate was presented by Mueller et al. [66] which handles and improve the activity of a sensor arrange. It explicitly smears SwissGate on home automation applications, for instance, estimating temperature, air circulation, and freshening control parameters. Bimschas et al. [67] target giving a scarce degree of acumen to doors by endowing them to implement submission programme. They recommend a middle-ware for the channel to suggest four potential administrations: bond transformation, demand stashing, insightful storing, and revelation.

One more work by Jong-Wan et al. [68] represent a sensor arrange framework involving a fundamental server and a few detecting servers going about as entryways and associating with various sensor systems. Utilizing system subordinate detecting servers as doors brings about high execution and equipment cost just as deprived versatility, assembling such a plan wasteful for some IoT applications. In an allied work introduced in [69], an attachment set up administration situated nonexclusive passage is proposed to give straightforward and quick arrangement of different outer sensor organize presentations. The door compromises a legitimate degree of compatibility by encouraging diverse sensor systems to cooperate. Be that as it may, the middleware introduced in their effort needs insight and works on the desktop, restricting its relevance to some IoT presentations. In a comparable endeavor, Guoqiang et al. [70] recommend a universally useful intelligent entryway. It gives pluggable design which empowers correspondence among various conventions, brought together outside interfaces fitting for malleable programming advancement, and malleable convention to decipher distinctive sensor information.

Accordingly, to replace verve and decrease the expense of intelligent home, Bian et al. [71] represent another kind of canny home governor framework, utilizing an Android supported Phone as a transitory home entryway rather than the conventional passage to home. The point of the effort is to naturally shut down the idle gadgets by anticipating client conduct. In an alternate application space, in [72] proposes a system of a smart IPv6 over Low force Wireless Personal Area Networks (6LoWPAN) outskirt switch that resolves on neighborhood selections of well-being circumstances employing a Hidden Markov Model.

In another work, Satyanarayanan et al. [73] recommends that mobile gadgets might exploit complex findings, for example, recognition of faces and language understanding to upsurge humanoid comprehension. In any case, confinements in using power and extended WAN expectancy are unsatisfactory. The creators at that point advise cloudlets that comprise of a PC with remote availability in the region of the cell phone. A base Virtual Machine (VM) that are propelled from the cloudlets and arranged utilizing intersection content from the cell phone with wanted submission. The VMs are intended to relocate starting with one cloudlet then onto the next to permit universality. The creators guarantee that presentations work quicker with its design because of poor latencies and complex preparing power. Nonetheless, the creators face difficulties with respect to long propelling occasions. In [74], Stantchev et al. represent the advantages of tri-level i.e., Fog based engineering for a shrewd health-care foundation from servitization and business perspective. In any case, they just spotlight on significant level structural displaying viewpoints and do not talk about genuine usage and test assessment of the administrations.

Despite the fact that endeavors of utilizing an entryway in IoT have been significantly extended as of late, there are just little enhancements towards acknowledging smart doors smoothed out explicitly for the human services area. The vast majority of the introduced endeavors centre on universally useful gateway structures which influences the knowledge level because of absence of data about the application area. A portion of these endeavors limit their degree of insight just for attachment and-play capacity, or modifiable to different spaces. Some others simply centre on explicit areas, for example, smart devices enabled home.

Existing commitments utilizing a door as a delegate among sensors and distributed storage, think about an insignificant job for gateway, for instance relating basic arrangement of constraints. In barely any circumstances, an entryway is utilized for area explicit purposes. Be that as it may, such stages neglect to fulfill the necessities of different spaces. In the medicinal services area, especially for remote well-being checking, an elevated level of dependability, accessibility and vigor is requested. In addition, security and protection issues are of basic significance. The reason for our shrewd gateway is to fulfill these space explicit necessities by modifying gateways for the health-care area and giving knowledge closer to patients.

As should be obvious that IoT's forthcoming is enhancing in the zones of medication, medicinal services, and well-being. In any case, it requests a shrewd biological system that will permit inter-connection amid all partners such as patients, doctors (in centers), enormous emergency clinics, urban areas and networks.

METHODS

The IoT empowered cloud computing framework is an IoT based distributed computing model for human services, which might deal with the information of people adequately, analyze and anticipate the wellbeing status to distinguish any illness. This system coordinates different hardware equipment through programming segments and permits organized and consistent start to finish reconciliation for quick and precise conveyance of outcomes.

Figure 1 depicts the architecture of IoT enabled cloud computing framework with various hardware and software modules that are described in section 3.1. The proposed models consist of training and testing models. The data acquired from doctors and experts are fed to the training model and their predicted results are stored in the cloud resource for testing the real-time from the persons. The training model accepts real-time data from various sensory devices and pre-processes them for computing. Since, the data acquired need not always be of computable form for the computing models to perform some operations with them.

The proposed model uses 'n' number of deep learning models as it always made possible because of the advancement in hardware resources and technology. These deep learning-based models along with the training sets of data checks the parameters in the acquired data. The prediction model gets expected results from various deep learning models and follows polling to choose the one of the following classes:

1) The patient with no disease.
2) The patient has a likelihood of getting disease.
3) The patient is predicted with disease.

IoT Enabled Cloud Computing Framework Components

The IoT enabled cloud computing framework consists of following components:

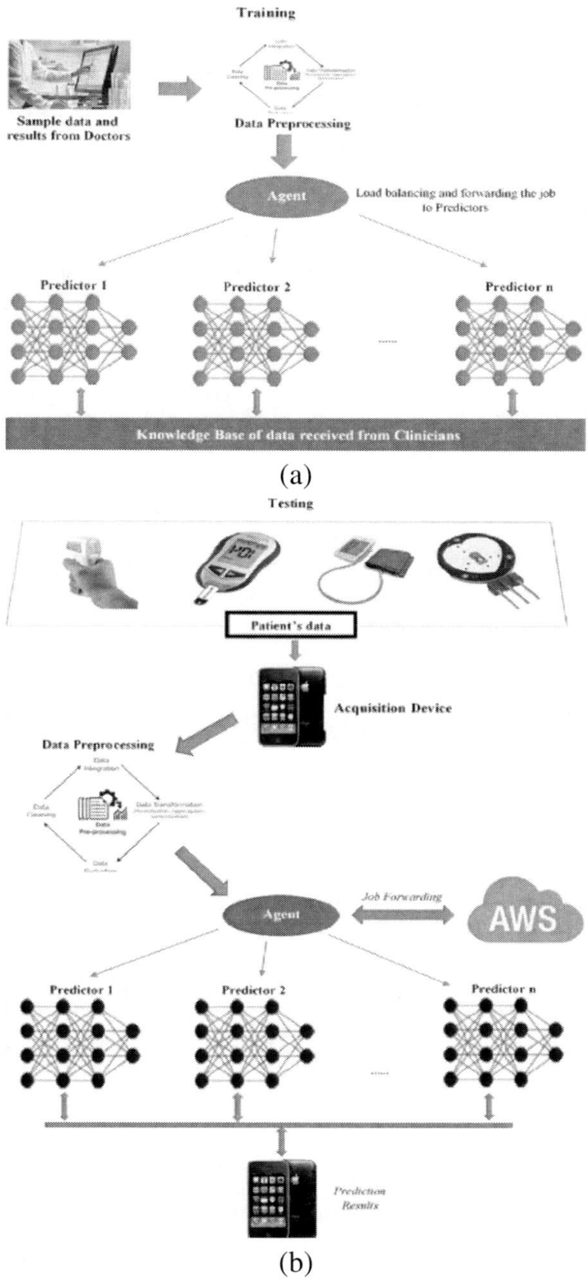

Figure 1(a) Training module & (b). Testing module.
The architecture of IoT enabled cloud computing framework.

Acquisition Device

The real-time data can be acquired from different types of sensors such as temperature sensor, pressure sensors, Electro Cardio Gram (ECG) sensor, Electro MyoGraphy (EMG) sensor, oxygen level sensor, sugar level sensor, inhalation rate sensor, glucose level sensor, Neural recording, Motion sensor, Physical activity sensor, wearable sensors and few off-Body sensors. This segment detects the information from people and moves to any of the associated gadgets like cell phones, PC and tablets which are going to act as a source to gather detected information from various sensors and forward this to different parts of the model for additional processing.

Pre-Processing Data

After acquiring input from your gadgets, the first and foremost step is to pre-process those inputs into some digital form which will be useful for the analyzer or the predictor to gather information for it. This incorporates information separating utilizing information examination devices. The sifted information is diminished to a littler measurement utilizing Principal Component Analysis (PCA) utilizing Set Partitioning in Hierarchical Trees (SPIHT) calculation [75] and encoded utilizing Singular Value Decomposition (SVD) strategy [76] with an objective of separating significant segments of information include directions that influence the patient's well-being status. In light of the removed information, it naturally settles on the choice, which suggests prescription and appropriate registration dependent on the persistent preparing information of medicinal services suppliers, specialists and stores in a database for reusing if required. The information got from basic ECG gadgets is an ordinary graph type pattern which should be pre-processed to discover estimations of numerous highlights of the contribution to the profound learning model [77, 78]. This requires application explicit space information to be taken care of into the framework.

An agent node is assigned in this model to do this pre-processing along with load balancing and resource managing. The load balancing keeps up work solicitation and undertaking lines for information preparing. It likewise handles majority of information which should be prepared. It plans the provisioned cloud assets for preparing of errands lined and kept up by the outstanding task at load balancer. The principle objective is to separate assignments to various gadgets to adjust the loads, give ideal execution and produce best outcomes. The proposed conspire permits clients to establish their own load adjustments and intervention plans dependent on the application prerequisites. The suggested scheme is defined as a flow graph in Figure 2.

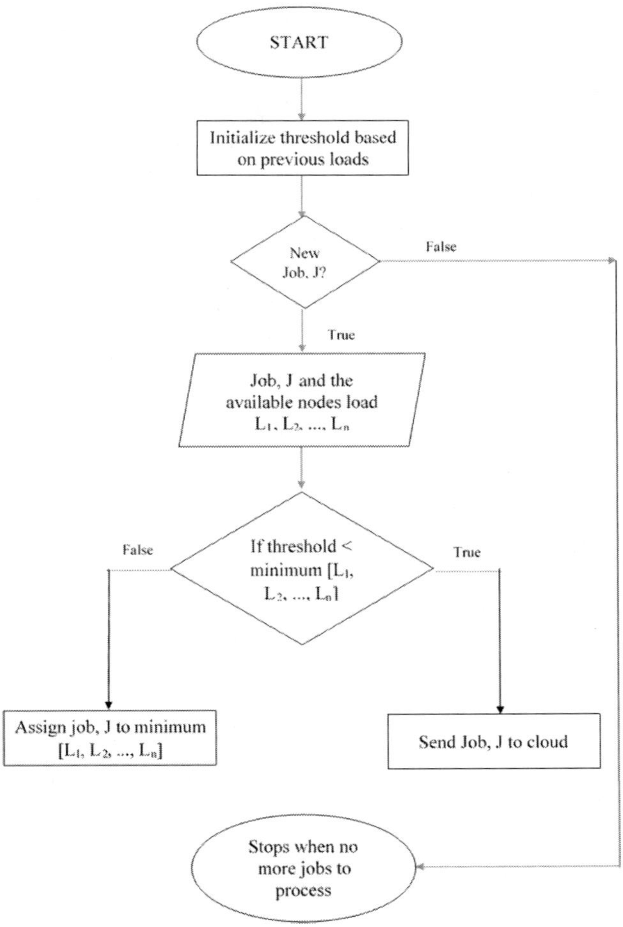

Figure 2. The proposed scheme for resource scheduling and load balancing.

Deep Learning Models

These models utilize the data sources to prepare a Neural Network in order to focus the highlight directions got after pre-processing the information acquired from the Sensors through the gadgets. In view of the errand allotted by agents, it additionally prophesies and produces outcomes for the information acquired from associated gadgets. This models additionally gets forecast outcomes from various representations and practices surveying to choose the either of the following classes: a) The patient with no disease, b) The patient has a likelihood of getting disease, c) The patient is predicted with disease. The profound neural system is utilized as a model for the prescient investigation, and for presentation the model is utilized for double order issue. The system model is initially prepared on the Electronic Health Record data source and comparing realized yield class and afterward the prepared system model is utilized for foreseeing consequences of constant information contribution as appeared in Figure 3.

We separate the information into training, validation and testing set in the proportion of 60:20:20. The training set is utilized for preparing the system, the validation set is utilized for regulating the model and the testing set is utilized for testing how the model executes on real-time information. The prepared system model can be put away in all the nodes equipped for handling by first putting away in a typical database. Other methodology will be to prepare system models independently by circulating the preparation data that focuses through various models. In appropriated preparing, information circulation utilizes procedures like boosting which haphazardly tests information from the data source with substitution and directs to various edge nodes for preparing singular system models.

At identification time, at whatever point a node is doled out an assignment, it gets the patients information in a vector of size 15. This information is taken care of as contribution to the system, creates an audacious authorization on the profound neural system and yields 1 or 0 for example regardless of the patient with illness or not. At analysis time, we utilize the collaborative technique for packing to consolidate the outcome of different models to give increasingly exact outcomes. The specialist that acquires the basic information multicasts it to other nodes. Every specialist at that point adds this to its line and the expectation consequences of every labor node are sent back to the specialist allocated for this errand. At that point the larger part expectation class acquired in by packing is sent it to the gateway gadget. We allow clients to cripple this element when the outcomes required are inertness basic.

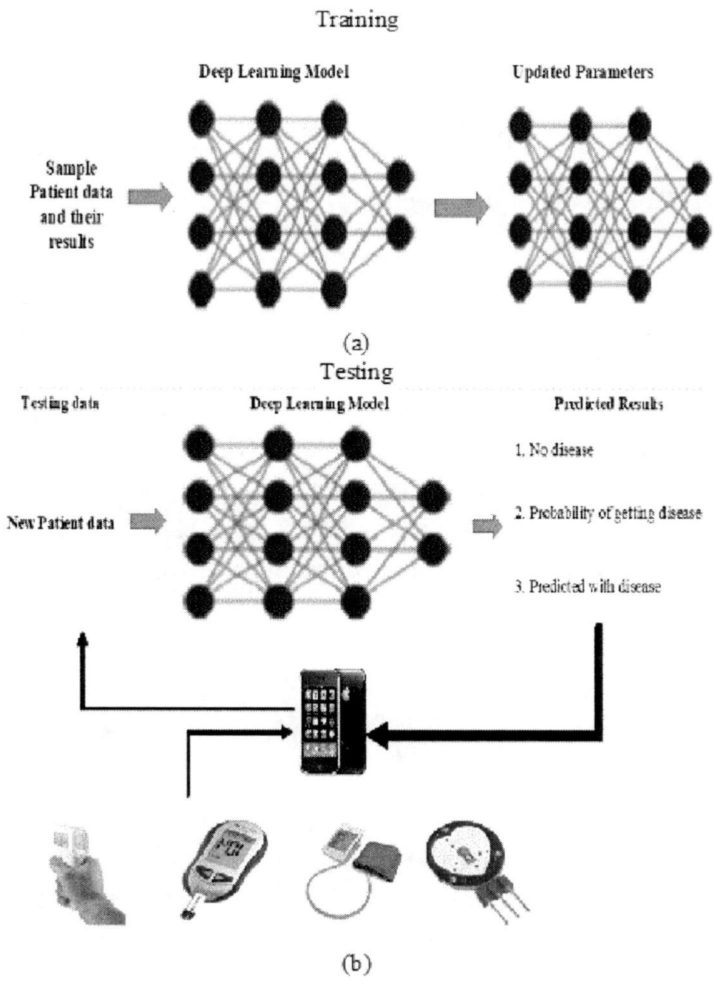

Figure 3(a) & (b). Training and Testing of the application.

The following are the attributes of the best underlying model on our data source after correction:

- Input layer's size: 15 (number of features of the data)
- Output layer's size: 3 (Trinity classification; a) The patient with no disease, b) The patient has a likelihood of getting disease, c) The patient is predicted with disease)
- Total hidden layers: 5 Layers
- Layer descriptions: Fully connected (FC) layer with 25 nodes
- Optimizer used: Adam
- Activation function used: Soft Max

Diagnose and Prediction Result

Data Source

These data incorporate measures for Electronic Health Record (EHR) reception, patient well-being data trade, including proportions of interoperable trade, and patient commitment abilities. The present review was handled from October 2017 as far as possible of February 2018. This review comprises of non-government, intense consideration clinics, including kids' and malignant growth medical clinics. This records for intense consideration general clinical and careful, general children's, and disease emergency clinics claimed by private/not-revenue driven, financial specialist owned/for-benefit, or state/neighborhood government and situated inside the 50 states and District of Columbia. The CEO of every clinic was welcome to take an interest in the study paying little mind to American Hospital Association (AHA) enrolment status. The individual generally learned about the emergency clinic's well-being IT (regularly the main data official) was mentioned to give the data by means of a mail overview or secure online website. Non-respondents got follow-up mailings and calls to support reaction. The table 1 speaks to the data field related with the dataset [86].

Table 1. Data field and their descriptions

Data Field	Data Description
region	Region - The region name for the data.
region_code	Region Code - The abbreviation code for the region name.
period	Time Period - Time period for the data. Year in which data was collected through survey. The first four digits correspond to the year of the data, and any other digits refer to the month of the data, beginning with "01"/January and ending with "12"/December.
pct_hospitals_basic_ ehr_notes	Percent of All Hospitals that have Adopted at least a Basic EHR with Clinician Notes - This measure estimates the percentage of all non-federal acute care hospitals that have adopted a basic EHR that is equipped with clinician notes.
pct_rural_hospitals_ basic_ehr_notes	Percent of Rural Hospitals that have Adopted at least a Basic EHR with Clinician Notes - This measure estimates the percentage of all rural non-federal acute care hospitals that have adopted a basic EHR that is equipped with clinician notes.
pct_small_hospitals_ basic_ehr_notes	Percent of Small Hospitals that have Adopted at least a Basic EHR with Clinician Notes - This measure estimates the percentage of all small non-federal acute care hospitals that have adopted a basic EHR that is equipped with clinician notes. A small hospital is defined as a facility with less than 100 inpatient beds.
pct_critical_access_hospitals_ basic_ehr_notes	Percent of Critical Access Hospitals that have Adopted at least a Basic EHR with Clinician Notes - This measure estimates the percentage of all non-federal acute care Critical Access hospitals that have adopted a basic EHR that is equipped with clinician notes.
pct_hospitals_basic_ ehr_no_notes	Percent of All Hospitals that have Adopted at least a Basic EHR without Clinician Notes - This measure estimates the percentage of all non-federal acute care hospitals that have adopted a basic EHR that is not equipped with clinician notes.
pct_rural_hospitals_basic_ ehr_no_notes	Percent of Rural Hospitals that have Adopted at least a Basic EHR without Clinician Notes - This measure estimates the percentage of all rural non-federal acute care hospitals that have adopted a basic EHR that is not equipped with clinician notes.
pct_small_hospitals_basic_ ehr_no_notes	Percent of Small Hospitals that have Adopted at least a Basic EHR without Clinician Notes - This measure estimates the percentage of all small non-federal acute care hospitals that have adopted a basic EHR that is not equipped with clinician notes. A small hospital is defined as a facility with less than 100 inpatient beds.

Table 1. (Continued)

Data Field	Data Description
pct_critical_access_hospitals_basic_ehr_no_notes	Percent of Critical Access Hospitals that have Adopted at least a Basic EHR without Clinician Notes - This measure estimates the percentage of all non-federal acute care Critical Access hospitals that have adopted a basic EHR that is not equipped with clinician notes.
pct_hospitals_cehrt	Percent of All Hospitals that have Adopted a Certified EHR - This measure estimates the percentage of all non-federal acute care hospitals that have adopted a certified EHR.
pct_small_rural_hospitals_cehrt	Percent of Small Rural Hospitals that have Adopted a Certified EHR - This measure estimates the percentage of all small rural non-federal acute care hospitals that have adopted a certified EHR.
pct_cah_hospitals_cehrt	Percent of Critical Access Hospitals that have Adopted a Certified EHR - This measure estimates the percentage of all Critical Access hospitals that have adopted a certified EHR.
pct_hospitals_share_labs_any_outside_provs	Percent of All Hospitals with Capability to Electronically Share Laboratory Results with Any Providers Outside their Health System - This measure estimates the percentage of all non-federal acute care hospitals that electronically exchange and/or share patient laboratory results with either hospitals or ambulatory providers outside the hospital's health system.
pct_hospitals_share_labs_any_outside_hospitals	Percent of All Hospitals with Capability to Electronically Share Laboratory Results with Hospitals Outside their Health System - This measure estimates the percentage of all non-federal acute care hospitals that electronically exchange and/or share patient laboratory results with hospitals outside the hospital's health system.
pct_hospitals_share_labs_any_outside_ambu_provs	Percent of All Hospitals with Capability to Electronically Share Laboratory Results with Ambulatory Providers Outside their Health System - This measure estimates the percentage of all non-federal acute care hospitals that electronically exchange and/or share patient laboratory results with ambulatory providers outside the hospital's health system.
pct_hospitals_patients_ecopy_ehr	Percent of All Hospitals with Capability to Provide Patients with an Electronic Copy of their EHR within 3 Business Days of the Request - This measure estimates the percentage of all non-federal acute care hospitals that have the capability to provide patients with an electronic copy of their electronic health record within three business days of the patient's request for the record.

Data Field	Data Description
pct_hospitals_patients_ecopy_ discharge_instr	Percent of All Hospitals with Capability to Provide Patients an Electronic Copy of their Discharge Instructions upon Request - This measure estimates the percentage of all non-federal acute care hospitals that have the capability to provide patients with an electronic copy of their discharge instructions upon the patient's request.
pct_hospitals_share_care_ summaries_any_ outside_provs	Percent of All Hospitals with Capability to Exchange Summary Care Record with Any Providers Outside their Health System - This measure estimates the percentage of all non-federal acute care hospitals that electronically exchange and/or share patient summary care records with either hospitals or ambulatory providers outside the hospital's health system.
pct_hospitals_share_care_ summaries_any_outside_ hospitals	Percent of All Hospitals with Capability to Exchange Summary Care Record with Hospitals Outside their Health System - This measure estimates the percentage of all non-federal acute care hospitals that electronically exchange and/or share patient summary care records with hospitals outside the hospital's health system.
pct_hospitals_share_care_ summaries_any_outside_ ambu_provs	Percent of All Hospitals with Capability to Exchange Summary Care Record with Ambulatory Providers Outside their Health System - This measure estimates the percentage of all non-federal acute care hospitals that electronically exchange and/or share patient summary care records with ambulatory providers outside the hospital's health system.
pct_hospitals_patients_vdt	Percent of All Hospitals with Capability for Patients to Electronically View, Download, and Transmit their Personal Health Information and Health Record - This measure estimates the percentage of all non-federal acute care hospitals that have the capability for their patients to electronically view, download, and transmit their personal health and medical information, as well as their health and medical record.
pct_hospitals_patients_ secure_message	Percent of All Hospitals with Capability for Patients to Securely Message with Providers - This measure estimates the percentage of all non-federal acute care hospitals that have the capability for their patients to securely message with their providers.
pct_hospitals_find_ clinical_info	Percent of All Hospitals that Electronically Find Patient Health Information from Outside Providers - This measure estimates the percentage of all hospitals that electronically find or query patient health information sources outside their organization or hospital system.
pct_hospitals_send_ clinical_info	Percent of All Hospitals that Electronically Send Patient Summary of Care Records to Outside Providers - This measure estimates the percentage of all hospitals that electronically send patient summary of care records to sources outside their organization or hospital system.

Table 1. (Continued)

Data Field	Data Description
pct_hospitals_receive_ clinical_info	Percent of All Hospitals that Electronically Receive Patient Summary of Care Records from Outside Providers - This measure estimates the percentage of all hospitals that electronically receive patient summary of care records to sources outside their organization or hospital system.
pct_hospitals_integrate_ any_clinical_info	Percent of All Hospitals that Electronically Integrate into an EHR Any Patient Information from Outside Providers - This measure estimates the percentage of all hospitals that integrate any patient information received electronically from sources outside their organization or hospital system without the need for manual entry.
pct_hospitals_integrate_scr	Percent of All Hospitals that Electronically Integrate into an EHR Patient Summary of Care Records from Outside Providers - This measure estimates the percentage of all hospitals that integrate summary of care records received electronically from sources outside their organization or hospital system without the need for manual entry.
pct_hospitals_send_ receive_find_integrate	Percent of All Hospitals that Electronically Send, Receive and Find Clinical Information and Integrate into an EHR Patient Summary of Care Records from Outside Providers - This measure estimates the percentage of all hospitals can send, receive and find clinical information from outside sources, and integrate a summary of care into an EHR without manual entry.
pct_hospitals_api	Percent of Hospitals that Provide their Patients the Ability to Access their Health Information Using an Application Programming Interface (API) - This measure estimates the percentage of hospitals that whose patients could access their health information using any application configured to meet the API specifications in the hospital's EHR.
pct_hospitals_integrate_pdmp	Percent of Hospitals that Can Access State Prescription Drug Monitoring Program (PDMP) within their EHR - This measure reports on the percent of hospitals, nationally and by state that responded that the hospital checks the state PDMP data within the hospital EHR system.

Utilizing the data source attributes referenced above, the system model is tested to see how fine it achieves to predict the patients with an illness or not on the estimations of the attributes indicated for every patient. The data source was separated into three segments of 60%, 20% and 20% of the entire information. The initial segment was utilized to prepare the model, the second for approval and tweaking the model attributes. The final part was utilized for testing the model execution. To quantify the presentation of the Cloud registering system, the accompanying attributes were watched and investigated:

1) *Prediction accuracies*: The dataset comprises of 1470 models in which 982 models were utilized for preparing the model and 488 models were utilized for testing. The preparation models were isolated similarly over all nodes similarly to get their separate prepared profound learning models. Since, the quantity of nodes increments to utilize all assets for preparing the data source models would need to be disseminated to all other nodes. This decreases the preparation time yet in addition the test exactness. To watch such impacts, the preparation and test exactness's were breaking down. We characterize precision all the more officially as the level of the complete patients for which the system model prophesies effectively in the event that they possess illness or not. We think about exactness's for various cloud settings, by fluctuating the quantity of nodes and with or without collaborating of outcomes.
2) *Time characteristics*: An agent subset of the distinctive planning attributes appeared in Figure 3 were likewise watched and contemplated. These incorporate intervention time, inertness, time for completion and restlessness. We look at these planning attributes for various cloud settings by choosing no nodes or single node or 2 nodes (without or with ensembling) or having a cloud just calculation framework.
3) *Network bandwidth usage:* As the situation for example agent just, workers or cloud and the quantity of worker nodes influence the system utilization this was concentrated to discover the system use in various cases. Like the analyses for control attributes, we think about the network transfer speed utilization for the distinctive situations. This was done to discover the reliance of data transfer capacity utilization with various designs that cloud computing system provides.

4) *Power consumption*: Vitality being a significant explanation of move from cloud to fog areas, we likewise considered the force utilization in various situations. In view of the force utilization examines and different trials depicted before we talk about how extraordinary Cloud figuring system setups can be utilized for different client and application necessities.

Cloud Resources

At the point when the fog foundation becomes overburden, administrations are inertness lenient or the information size is a lot bigger than normal size, at that point distributed computing system bridles assets of Cloud Data Centers (CDC). This makes it increasingly powerful, fit for performing substantial burden errands rapidly and furthermore makes information preparing area free.

RESULTS AND DISCUSSION

The framework arrangement for the IoT empower cloud computing system assessment and the equipment designs are depicted beneath:

- *Mobile Device*: Samsung Galaxy S10 with android 10
- *Head Node*: HP Elite Dragonfly Notebook with Intel® Core™ i5-8365U, 16GB RAM, OS Recovery and Intel® UHD Graphics 620 with 64-bit Windows 10 Operating system and Apache HTTP Server 2.4.42
- *Other Node*: Raspberry Pi 4, Broadcom BCM2711, Quad core Cortex-A72 (ARM v8) 64-bit SoC @ 1.5GHz, 2GB LPDDR4-3200 SDRAM, Broadcom BCM2711, Quad core Cortex-A72 (ARM v8) 64-bit SoC @ 1.5GHz with Raspberry pi Operating system
- *Public Cloud*: Microsoft Azure B1s Machine, 1vCPU, 1GB RAM, 2GB SSD, Windows Server 2016.

Throughout the experimentations, result considerations are recorded at the head node using Microsoft Performance Monitor and the Azure VM whereas at the Raspberry Pi circuits NMON Performance Monitor is used [79, 80]. Head node [81] and the vnStat [82] tool in Raspberry Pis was used to quantity the network bandwidth consumption.

Prediction Accuracies

Figure 4 displays the comparison of training precision with increasing number of nodes. The training precision continuously increments as the quantity of nodes increments. In light of the fact that each node learns a model for the information obtained by it, and as the amount of node raises up, the number of models obtained by each node gets lesser and, in this way, preparing the model for various iterations over-fit the examples and thus training precision increments.

Figure 5 shows the comparison of test data precision with increasing number of nodes. True to form, test precision diminishes with increased number of nodes since every node gets a fewer subset of training information and henceforth cannot simplify the system. Additional perception is that, 'with collaborative' learning model consistently contributes much preferred precision over the 'without collaborative' learning model.

Timing Features

Figure 6 represents the comparison of intercession time at the node for diverse circumstances: (1) Head node, (2) Single node, (3) Two nodes, (4) Two nodes (collaborative), and (5) Cloud. We see that intercession time is nearly insignificant if the job is directly sent to Head node or Cloud. As the quantity of edge nodes raises, the head node prerequisites to check the loads at each other node and locate the least load node to send job, henceforth the intercession time raises as number of nodes raises. At the point when the information is sent to other node for collaborative learning, at that point additionally the head does not have to ensure any load scrutiny, as dominant part class decision should be finished by one of the nodes. In this way intercession time is more or less same as without collaborating case.

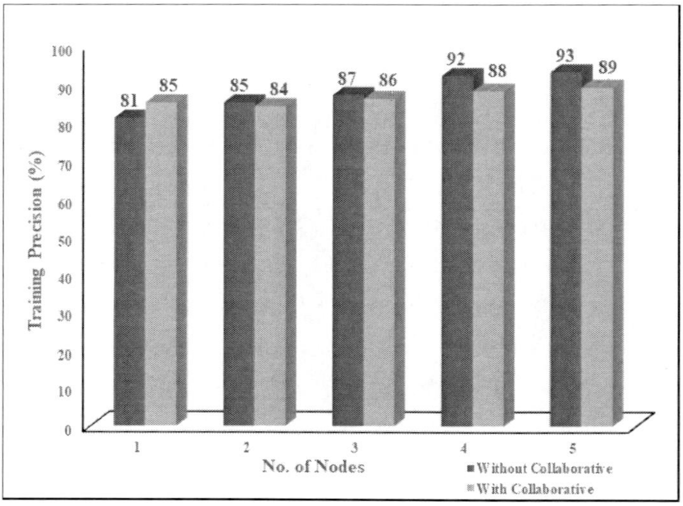

Figure 4. The comparison of training precision with increasing number of nodes.

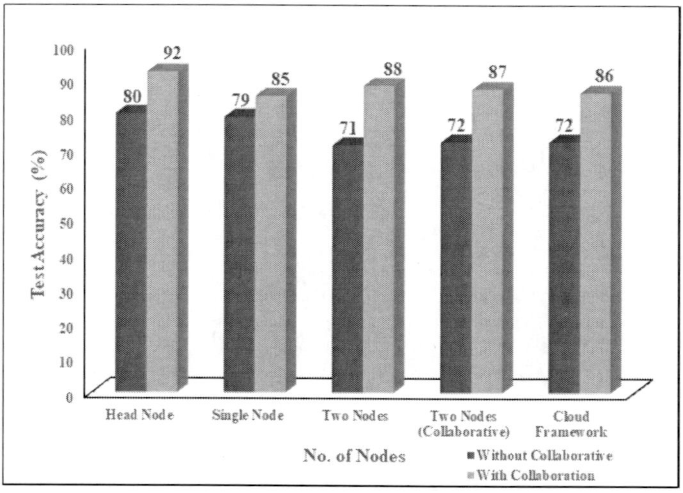

Figure 5. The comparison of test precision with increasing number of nodes.

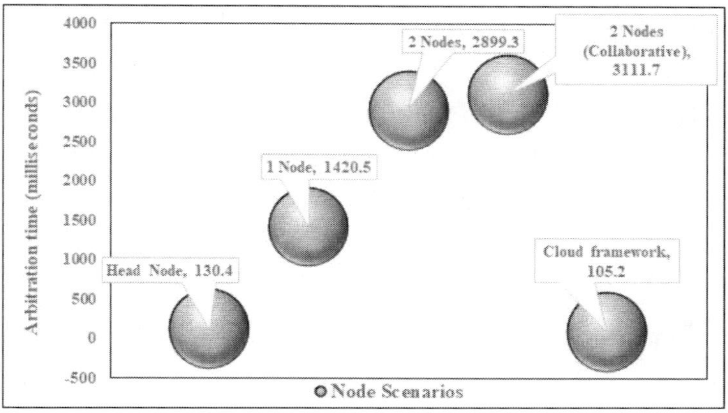

Figure 6. The comparison of intercession time at the node for different scenarios.

Figure 7 shows the comparison of latency at the node for different circumstances. If the assignment is sent to head or any of the other nodes, at that point the latency is about same as all correspondence is done solitary bounce information moves. In collaborative case, the latency is higher to a certain extent. In arrears to multi-bounce exchange of information outside the LAN, the latency is extremely high for cloud setting.

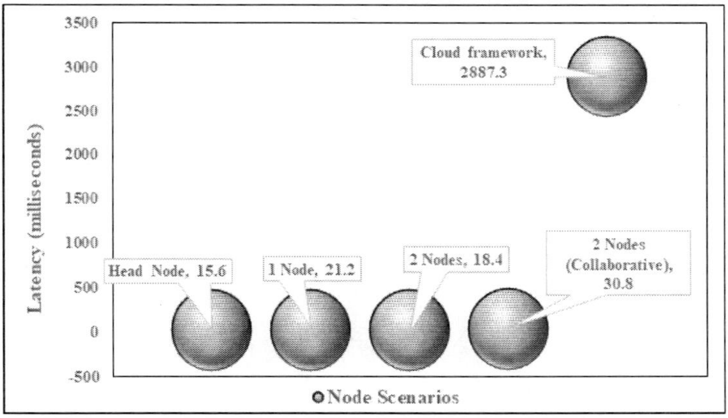

Figure 7. The comparison of latency at the node for different scenarios.

Network Bandwidth Usage

Figure 8 shows the comparison of Network bandwidth usage of all nodes in diverse circumstances. As the number of other nodes increase, the handling of network bandwidth also raises as extra new data packets, safety authorizations and data assignment including relocation to cloud are necessary. As data is guided to all raspberry nodes, network bandwidth utilization is most elevated in collaborative case.

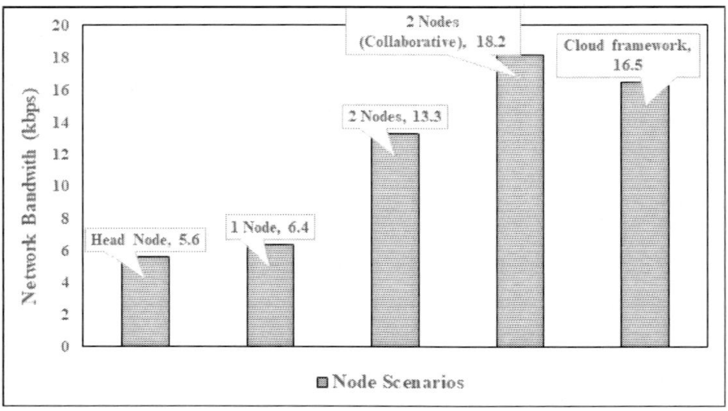

Figure 8. The comparison of Network bandwidth usage of all nodes in diverse node consequences.

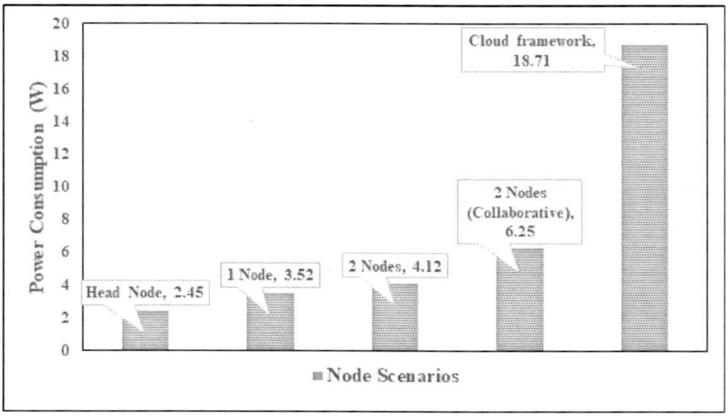

Figure 9. The tested power consumption characteristics in different node scenarios.

Power Characteristics

Figure 9 shows the tested power consumption characteristics in diverse node consequences. The CDC's power consumption is extremely high when compared with the head node (PC) or other node (Raspberry Pi) that prompts extremely large power consumption in other case contrasted with cloud case. As the quantity of raspberry nodes raises, the power consumption of Automatic Healthcare system likewise increments.

Through the progression of deep learning-based forecast system models, smart health care framework can utilize best in classical Neural Network models for exceptionally exact expectation of features of patient's health. Different works like [22, 35] come up short on the capacity to coordinate such system models and subsequently give minor illness discovery precision and is pivotal to give low latency and profoundly precise outcomes in basic healthcare applications particularly those worried about diabetes, lung disease, epidermal disease, pandemic disease, heart disease and cancer related issues. Moreover, works that utilization deep learning [83, 84, and 85] do not utilize collaborating techniques to give far and away superior outcomes by utilizing cloud assets for equal calculation and giving fundamentally higher precision. As appeared by results about Section 4.1, the prediction accuracy along with collaborating increments by 20% for the case with 2 nodes which is essentially greater than what prevailing frameworks (without collaborative deep learning) could contribute.

The work built up a latency and precision considering use of patient examination utilizing the cloud-based structure with straightforwardness and in low time to productively utilize cloud assets. The application organization framework gave various arrangements that give better precision or latency dependent on client prerequisites. In view of the exploratory outcomes, we propose IoT empowered cloud computing system to be developed in the following backgrounds dependent on the objective applications:

- For unconsciousness acute and frivolous errands or power constraints conditions, nodes ought to be utilized. This gives stumpy results conveyance time because of the closeness of raspberry nodes. In the event that energy and network bandwidth limitations exist, at that point collaborative clustering ought to be weakened. Yet if not, empowering collaborative would bring in best precision.
- For substantial and latency lenient errands, CDC arrangement might be utilized in any case such undertakings would not have the possibility to effectively finish on resource limitation edge raspberry nodes.

CONCLUSION

The IoT enabled cloud computing framework discuss the significant areas of health-care such as epidemic diseases, pandemic diseases, heart diseases, respiratory diseases, diabetes, hepatitis and cancer, which can afford skilled facilities to supportive patients. In this work, a novel intelligent healthcare system for automatic diagnosis of diseases using deep learning and IoT enabled cloud computing framework is proposed targeting on the healthcare facets for patients. The framework efficiently handles the data from patients received from different IoT devices and supplies e-healthcare as a facility. Despite the merits obtainable by IoT, many encounters must to be embarked upon such as scalability, data administration, interoperability, safety and secrecy and device-network human interfaces. It assimilates and deploys deep learning for disease analysis through a real-life application. Preceding mechanisms on similar patient data investigations never employed deep learning so it had week prediction precision which makes them unserviceable in practical environments. Deep learning-based representations with extremely high precision involve exceedingly high computing properties for both training and testing. The proposed work permitted multifaceted deep learning networks to be entrenched in cloud computing prototypes with innovative communication and typical dissemination methods like collaborating which permitted high precision to be accomplished with remarkably low latencies. The framework was also authenticated for real-time patient data investigation by training neural networks on standard data sets and installing an operational structure that contributes prediction outcomes in real-time. A cloud framework is used to corroborate the system and to test the effectiveness of suggested system in terms of training precision, testing precision, latency time, intercession time, power consumption characteristics and network bandwidth.

As a segment of future effort, there is plan to recommend the approach to certificate cost-ideal implementation given diverse QoS qualities and cloud rate models. Increasingly insightful collaborative system models will be conveyed for added augmenting the exactness. Further, the projected design can be built more powerful and nonexclusive to combine further distributed computing presentations, for example, farming, tele-medicine, climate estimating, smart building, and smart cities with traffic monitoring.

References

[1] Gubbi J, Buyya R, Marusic S, and Palaniswami M. 2013. "Internet of things (IoT): A vision, architectural elements, and future directions." *Future Generation Computer Systems* 29(7):1645–1660.

[2] Atzori L, Iera A, and Morabito G. 2010. "The internet of things: A survey." *Computer networks* 54(15):2787–2805.

[3] Vilamovska AM, Hatziandreu E, Schindler HR, Van Oranje-Nassau C, de Vries H, and Krapels J. 2009. "Study on the requirements and options for RFID application in healthcare." *Scoping and Identifying areas for Radio Frequency Identification deployment in healthcare delivery: a review of relevant literature*. Directorate General Information Society and Media, European Commission. Santa Monica, CA, USA: The RAND Corporation.

[4] Alemdar H, and Ersoy C. 2010. “Wireless sensor networks for healthcare: A survey.” *Computer Networks* 54(15):2688–2710.

[5] Farahani BJ, and Fathy M. 2009. “Improving coverage in mobile sensor networks using overlap concept.” in *CSI Computer Conference, 2009. CSICC 2009. 14th International CSI*633–639.

[6] Farahani BJ, Ghaffarian H, and Fathy M. 2010. “A fuzzy based priority approach in mobile sensor network coverage.” *ACEEE International Journal of Network Security* 1(2):45–50.

[7] Soleimanzadeh R, Farahani BJ, and Fathy M. 2010. “PSO based deployment algorithms in hybrid sensor networks.” *Computer Science*.

[8] Soleimanzadeh R, Farahani BJ, Fathy M et al. 2010. “Improved dynamic k-coverage algorithms in mobile sensor networks.” *Wireless Sensor Network* 2(10):784-792.

[9] Saravi M and Farahani BJ. 2009. “*Distance Constrained Deployment (DCD) algorithm in mobile sensor networks*.” presented at Third International Conference on Next Generation Mobile Applications, Services and Technologies, 435–440.

[10] Da Xu L, He W, and Li S. 2014. “Internet of things in industries: A survey,” *Industrial Informatics, IEEE Transactions on*, 10(4):2233–2243.

[11] Welbourne E, Battle L, Cole G, Gould K, Rector K, Raymer S, Balazinska M, and Borriello G. 2009. “Building the internet of things using RFID: the RFID ecosystem experience.” *Internet Computing, IEEE* 13(3):48–55.

[12] Miorandi D, Sicarib S, De Pellegrini F, and Chlamtac I. 2012. “Internet of things: Vision, applications and research challenges,” *Ad Hoc Networks* 10(7):1497–1516.

[13] Bandyopadhyay D and Sen J. 2011. “Internet of things: Applications and challenges in technology and standardization.” *Wireless Personal Communications*, 58(1):49–69.

[14] Sundmaeker H, Guillemin P, Friess P, and Woelffle S. 2010. “Vision and challenges for realising the internet of things.” *European commission information society and media*. 89-189.

[15] Haller S., Karnouskos S., Schroth C. 2009. "The Internet of Things in an Enterprise Context." In: Domingue J., Fensel D., Traverso P. (eds.) *Future Internet – FIS 2008. FIS 2008.* Lecture Notes in Computer Science, Springer, Berlin, Heidelberg, 5468.

[16] Zheng Z, Zhu J, and Lyu MR. 2013. "Service-generated big data and big data-as-a-service: an overview," *presented in Big Data (Big Data Congress), 2013 IEEE International Congress on. IEEE*403–410.

[17] Keim DA, Kohlhammer J, Ellis G, and Mansmann F. 2010. "Mastering the information age: solving problems with visual analytics." *Florian Mansmann.*

[18] Kim J. 2018. The Effect of Patient Participation through Physician's Resources on Experience and Well-being. *Sustainability* 10, 2102.

[19] Aloqaily M, Kantarci B, Mouftah. 2016. "Multiagent /multiobjective interaction game system for service provisioning in vehicular cloud." *IEEE Access* 4:3153–3168.

[20] Kuo MHA. 2016. "Opportunities and Challenges of Cloud Computing to Improve Health Care Services." *J. Med. Internet Res.* 13, e67.

[21] Otoum S, Ahmed M, Mouftah HT. 2015. "Sensor Medium Access Control (SMAC)-based epilepsy patients monitoring system." In *Proceedings of the 2015 IEEE 28th Canadian Conference on Electrical and Computer Engineering (CCECE),* Halifax, NS, Canada. 3(6):1109–1114.

[22] Gia TN, Jiang M, Rahmani AM, Westerlund T, Liljeberg P, Tenhunen H. 2015. "Fog Computing in Healthcare Internet of Things: A Case Study on ECG Feature Extraction." In *Proceedings of the 2015 IEEE International Conference on Computer and Information Technology; Ubiquitous Computing and Communications; Dependable, Autonomic and Secure Computing; Pervasive Intelligence and Computing,* Liverpool, UK. 26(28):356–363.

[23] Esposito M, Minutolo A, Megna R, Forastiere M, Magliulo M, Pietro, GD. 2018. "A smart mobile, self-configuring, context-aware

architecture for personal health monitoring." *Eng. Appl. Artif. Intell.* 67:136–156.

[24] Salama U, Yao L, Paik HY. 2018. "An Internet of Things Based Multi-Level Privacy-Preserving Access Control for Smart Living." *Informatics*, 5(23):1-18.

[25] Taherizadeh S, Stankovski V, Grobelnik M. 2018. "A Capillary Computing Architecture for Dynamic Internet of Things: Orchestration of Microservices from Edge Devices to Fog and Cloud Providers." *Sensors*, 18:29-38.

[26] Shah SA, Ren A, Fan D, Zhang Z, Zhao N, Yang X, Luo M, Wang W, HuF, Rehman MU, et al. 2018. "Internet of Things for Sensing: A Case Study in the Healthcare System." *Appl. Sci.* 8, 508.

[27] Sodhro AH, Sangaiah AK, Sodhro GH, Lohano S, Pirbhulal S. 2018. "An Energy-Efficient Algorithm for Wearable Electrocardiogram Signal Processing in Ubiquitous Healthcare Applications." *Sensors* 18, 923.

[28] Hossain M, Islam SR, Ali F, Kwak KS, Hasan R. 2018. "An Internet of Things-based health prescription, assistant and its security system design." *Future Gener. Comput. Syst.* 82:422–439.

[29] Zeng Z, Ma X, Hu Y, Li J, Bryant D. 2012. "A simulation study to improve quality of care in the emergency department of a community hospital." *J. Emerg. Nurs.* 38: 322–328.

[30] Aloqaily M, Kantarci B, Mouftah HT. 2014. "On the impact of quality of experience (QoE) in a vehicular cloud with various providers." In *Proceedings of the 2014 11th Annual High Capacity Optical Networks and Emerging/Enabling Technologies (Photonics for Energy),* Charlotte, NC, USA 15(17):94–98.

[31] Buckley BJ, Castillo EM, Killeen JP, Guss DA, Chan TC. 2010. "Impact of an express admit unit on emergency department length of stay." *J. Emerg. Med.* 39:669–673.

[32] Soremekun OA, Takayesu JK, Bohan SJ. 2011. "Framework for analyzing wait times and other factors that impact patient satisfaction in the emergency department." *J. Emerg. Med.* 41:686–692.

[33] Alvarez AM, Centeno MA. 1999. "Enhancing simulation models for emergency rooms using VBA." In *Proceedings of the 1999Winter Simulation Conference Proceedings,* Phoenix, AZ, USA2:1685–1693.

[34] Islam SMR, Kwak D, Kabir MDH, Hossain M and Kwak KS. 2015. "The internet of things for health care: a comprehensive survey." *IEEE Access*. 3:678-708.

[35] Rahmani AM, Gia TN, Negash B, Anzanpour A, Azimi I, Jiang M, and Liljeberg P. 2018. "Exploiting smart e-health gateways at the edge of healthcare internet-of-things: A fog computing approach." *Future Generation Computer Systems* 78:641-658.

[36] Goyal, Abhishek, Kanika Narang, Gautam Ahluwalia, Sohal PM, Bhupinder Singh, Shibba T. Chhabra, Naved Aslam, Bishav Mohan, and Gurpreet S. Wander. 2019. "Seasonal variation in 24h blood pressure profile in healthy adults-A prospective observational study." *Journal of human hypertension* 1:2019.

[37] Mutlag, Ammar Awad, Mohd Khanapi Abd Ghani, Net al Arunkumar, Mazin Abed Mohamed, and Othman Mohd. 2019. "Enabling technologies for fog computing in healthcare IoT systems." *Future Generation Computer Systems* 90: 62-78.

[38] Gill, Sukhpal Singh, Peter Garraghan, and Rajkumar Buyya. 2019. "ROUTER: Fog enabled cloud based intelligent resource management approach for smart home IoT devices." *Journal of Systems and Software* 154:125-138.

[39] Faust, Oliver, Yuki Hagiwara, Tan Jen Hong, Oh ShuLih, and U. Rajendra Acharya. 2018. "Deep learning for healthcare applications based on physiological signals: A review" *Computer methods and programs in biomedicine* 161:1-13.

[40] Tuli, Shreshth, Nipam Basumatary and Rajkumar Buyya. 2019. "Edgelens: Deep learning-based object detection in integrated IoT, fog and cloud computing environments." *Proceedings of the 4th IEEE International Conference on Information Systems and Computer Networks (ISCON 2019, IEEE Press, USA),* Mathura, India, November 21-22.

[41] Dietterich, Thomas G. 2000. "Ensemble methods in machine learning." *In International workshop on multiple classifier systems, Springer, Berlin, Heidelberg* 1-15.

[42] Zhao, Xianlong, Kexin Yang, Qimei Chen, Duo Peng, Hao Jiang, Xianze Xu, and Xinzhuo Shuang. 2019. "Deep learning based mobile data offloading in mobile edge computing systems." *Future Generation Computer Systems*, 99:346-355.

[43] Lim, Tjen-Sien, Wei-Yin Loh, and Yu-Shan Shih. 2000. "A comparison of pre- diction accuracy, complexity, and training time of thirty-three old and new classification algorithms." *Machine learning* 40(3):203-228.

[44] Gill, Sukhpal Singh, Rajesh Chand Arya, Gurpreet Singh Wander, and Rajkumar Buyya. 2018. "Fog-Based Smart Healthcare as a Big Data and Cloud Service for Heart Patients Using IoT." In *International Conference on Intelligent Data Communication Technologies and Internet of Things, Springer,* Cham 376-1383.

[45] Sokol MC, McGuigan KA, Verbrugge RR, and Epstein RS. 2005. "Impact of medication adherence on hospitalization risk and healthcare cost." *Medical care,* 43(6):521–530.

[46] D. o. E. United Nations and P. D. Social Affairs. 2013. "World population ageing," *Computer Networks.*

[47] "Bulletin of the world health organization," *Computer Networks* 88(4):241–320, 2010.

[48] D. Association et al. 2013. "Economic costs of diabetes in the US in 2012. Diabetes care 2013; 36: 1033–1046." *Diabetes care,* 36(6):1797.

[49] Corrigan JM, Swift EK, Hurtado MP et al. 2001. "Envisioning the national health care quality report." *National Academies Press.*

[50] Hill CF, Powers BW, Jain SH, Bennet J, Vavasis A, and Oriol NE. 2014. "Mobile health clinics in the era of reform." *The American journal of managed care*, 20(3):261–264.

[51] Intelligence M. 2015. *Global Telemedicine Market Growth, Trends and Forecasts (2015-2019).* Available at http: www.mordor

intelligence.com/industryreports/global-telemedicine-market industry.

[52] Rashidi P and Mihailidis A. 2013. "A survey on ambient-assisted living tools for older adults," *Biomedical and Health Informatics, IEEE Journal of,* 17(3):579–590.

[53] Sadri F, 2011. "Ambient intelligence: A survey," *ACM Computing Surveys (CSUR)* 43(4):36.

[54] Aarts E and Encarnacao J. 2006. "*The emergence of ambient intelligence*." Berlin, Germany: Springer.

[55] Wang M, Zhang G, Zhang C, Zhang J, and Li C. 2013. "An IoT-based appliance control system for smart homes." In *Intelligent Control and Information Processing (ICICIP), 2013 Fourth International Conference on. IEEE* 744–747.

[56] Chourabi H, Nam T, Walker S, Gil-Garcia JR, Mellouli S, Nahon K, Pardo TA, and Scholl HJ. 2012. "Understanding smart cities: An integrative framework." *in System Science (HICSS), 2012 45th Hawaii International Conference on. IEEE*, 2289–2297.

[57] Harrison C, Eckman B, Hamilton R, Hartswick P, Kalagnanam J, Paraszczak J, and Williams P. 2010. "Foundations for smarter cities." *IBM Journal of Research and Development* 54(4):1–16.

[58] Sun Y, Song H, Jara AJ, and Bie R. 2016. "Internet of things and big data analytics for smart and connected communities," *IEEE Access* 4:766–773.

[59] Rathore MM, Paul A, Ahmad A, and Rho S. 2016. "Urban planning and building smart cities based on the internet of things using big data analytics." *Computer Networks*.

[60] N. S. Foundation, "*Supporting research advances in smart and connected communities*."

[61] Pla MAM, Lemus-Zúñiga LG, Montañana JM, Pons J, and Garza AA. 2016. "A review of mobile apps for improving quality of life of asthmatic and people with allergies." In *Innovation in Medicine and Healthcare 2015. Springer* 51–64.

[62] Lambrechts J and Sinha S. 2016. "Tools and facilitators towards successful planning for sustainable cities." *in Micro sensing Networks for Sustainable Cities. Springer* 269–305.

[63] Djahel S, Salehie M, Tal I, and Jamshidi P. 2013. "Adaptive traffic management for secure and efficient emergency services in smart cities," *in Pervasive Computing and Communications Workshops (PERCOM Workshops), 2013 IEEE International Conference on. IEEE*, 340–343.

[64] Emara KA, Abdeen M, and Hashem M. 2009. "A gateway-based framework for transparent interconnection between WSN and IP network." *In Proceedings of the EUROCON,* 1775-1780.

[65] Zhu Q, Wang R, Chen Q, Liu Y, and Qin W. 2010. "IoT Gateway: Bridging Wireless Sensor Networks into Internet of Things." In *Proceedings of the International Conference on Embedded and Ubiquitous Computing* 347-352.

[66] Mueller R, Rellermeyer JS, Duller M, and Alonso G. 2007. "Demo: A Generic Platform for Sensor Network Applications." In *Proceedings of the IEEE International Conference on Mobile Adhoc and Sensor Systems* 1-3.

[67] Bimschas D, Hellbruck H, Mietz R, Pfisterer D, Romer K, and Teubler T. 2010. "Middleware for Smart Gateways Connecting Sensornets to the Internet." In *Proceedings of the International Workshop on Middleware Tools, Services and Run-Time Support for Sensor Networks*8-14.

[68] Yoon JW, Ku YK, Nam CS, and Shin DR. 2009. "Sensor Network Middleware for Distributed and Heterogeneous Environments." In *Proceedings of the International Conference on New Trends in Information and Service Science* 979-982.

[69] Wu L, Xu Y, Xu C, and Wang F. 2013. "Plug-configure-play service-oriented gateway - for fast and easy sensor network application development." In *Proceedings of the International Conference on Sensor Networks*53-58.

[70] Guoqiang S, Yanming C, Chao Z, and Yanxu Z. 2013. "Design and Implementation of a Smart IoT Gateway." In *Proceedings of the*

International Conference on Green Computing and Communications and IEEE Internet of Things and IEEE Cyber, Physical and Social Computing 720-723.

[71] Bian J, Fan D, and Zhang J. 2011. "The new intelligent home control system based on the dynamic and intelligent gateway." In *Proceedings of the International Conference on Broadband Network and Multimedia Technology*, 526-530.

[72] Shen W, Xu Y, Xie D, Zhang T, and Johansson A. 2011. "Smart Border Routers for eHealth Care Wireless Sensor Networks." In *Proceedings of the International Conference on Wireless Communications, Networking and Mobile Computing* 1-4.

[73] Satyanarayanan M, Bahl P, Caceres R, and Davies N. 2009. "The Case for VM-Based Cloudlets in Mobile Computing." *IEEE Pervasive Computing* 8(4):14-23.

[74] Vladimir Stantchev, Ahmed Barnawi, Sarfaraz Ghulam, Johannes Schubert, and Gerrit Tamm. 2015. "Smart items, fog and cloud computing as enablers of servitization in healthcare." *Sensors & Transducers* 185(2):121.

[75] Hsieh JH, Lee RC, Hung KC, and Shih MJ. 2018. "Rapid and coding- efficient SPIHT algorithm for wavelet-based EC, data compression." *Integration, the VLSI Journal*, 60:248-256.

[76] Liu TY, Lin KY and Wu HC. 2017. "ECG Data Encryption Then Compression Using Singular Value Decomposition." *IEEE journal of biomedical and health informatics*.

[77] Kato, Norihiro, Marie Loh, Fumihiko Takeuchi, Niek Verweij, Xu Wang, Weihua Zhang, Tanika N. Kelly et al. 2015. "Trans-ancestry genome-wide association study identifies 12 genetic loci influencing blood pressure and implicates a role for DNA methylation." *Nature genetics* 47(11):1282.

[78] Sanghera, Dharambir K, Latonya Been, Lyda Ortega, Gurpreet S. Wan- der, Narinder K. Mehra, Christopher E. Aston, John J. Mulvihill, and SarjuRalhan. 2009. "Testing the association of novel meta-analysis-derived diabetes risk genes with type II diabetes and

related metabolic traits in Asian Indian Sikhs." *Journal of human genetics* 54(3):162.

[79] *Mircosoft Windows performance toolkit*. https:-docs.microsoft.com/en-us/windows-hardware/test/wpt/ [Online; accessed 28-March-2020].

[80] *SplunkBase performance monitor*. https:-splunkbase.splunk.com/app/1753/. [Online; accessed 28-March-2020].

[81] *Microsoft Network Monitor* 3.4. https:-www.microsoft.com/en-au/download/details.aspx?id=4865. [Online; accessed 28-March-2020].

[82] *vnStat Network monitoring tool*. https:-humdi.net/vnstat/. [Online; accessed 28-March-2020].

[83] Choi, Edward, Mohammad Taha Bahadori, Le Song, Walter F. Stewart, and Jimeng Sun. 2017. "GRAM: graph-based attention model for healthcare representation learning." In *Proceedings of the 23rd ACM SIGKDD International Conference on Knowledge Discovery and Data Mining*, 787-795.

[84] Constant, Nicholas, Debanjan Borthakur, Mohammadreza Abtahi, Harish chandra Dubey, and Kunal Mankodiya. 2017. "Fog-assisted WIoT: A smart fog gateway for end-to-end analytics in wearable internet of things." *arXiv preprint arXiv*: 1701.08680.

[85] Li, Liangzhi, Kaoru Ota, and Mianxiong Dong. 2018. "Deep learning for smart industry: efficient manufacture inspection system with fog computing." *IEEE Transactions on Industrial Informatics* 14(10): 4665-4673.

[86] *Non-federal Acute Care Hospital Health IT Adoption and Use*. https://dashboard.healthit.gov/datadashboard/documentation/hospital-health-it-adoption-use-data-documentation.php. [Online; accessed 28-March-2020].

In: Computing Paradigms for Smart Healthcare ISBN: 978-1-53618-619-2
Editors: B. Vinoth Kumar et al.

Chapter 4

Digital Twin Technology for Smart Health Care

M. S. Sangeetha*[*], PhD
Biomedical Engineering, PSG College of Technology,
Coimbatore, Tamil Nadu, India

Abstract

Digital twin technology is to develop a dynamic virtual representation of a system or a device using the advancements of computing techniques and Internet of Things. This technology is said to drive Industry 4.0 and revolutionize the developments in cyber physical systems across the globe. The advent of digital twin technology has led to reduced power, cost and increased productivity in the product development of various automotive and manufacturing industries. Digital twin technology has emerged in the healthcare industry in various domains to identify potential problems that may arise in the hospital system or equipment. Digital twins aid to prevent, maintain and predict the failures and for smart analysis of the healthcare system. The advancements in Artificial Intelligence and high-end computing

[*] Corresponding Author's Email: sangeetms@gmail.com.

algorithms, paves way towards a smarter patient-centric health care system. This chapter introduces the basic concepts of digital twin technology and implementation of digital twin in various health care domains.

Keywords: Digital Twin, Artificial Intelligence, Internet of Things, Cyber physical system

INTRODUCTION

As Industry 4.0 is gaining momentum globally, its main objective is to adopt new technologies such as Data analytics and Internet –of –Things (IoT) to enhance its competitiveness. The advancements of computing paradigms have led to the broad spectrum of industrial verticals. The purpose of the Digital Twin technology is to create a virtual representation of the physical object in the real world, facilitated by IoT platforms and software. The digital equivalent to a physical product or the Digital Twin has evolved as the standard feature which could be incorporated into the IoT platforms for product lifecycle management. The virtually created object can be used to manipulate and control the real-world item, which seems to be the vision of the Industrial 4.0 to digitize the products. The role of Digital Twin (DT) has emerged in the healthcare industry to revolutionize the concept of personalized medicine. The digital replica of the healthcare equipment or asset or the individual human is created from the physical entities in order to achieve specific clinical and economic goals of the health care system.

This chapter provides an insight about the role of Digital twin in healthcare, its conceptual architecture, recent trends in Digital Twin Technology (DTT) and the challenges and solutions for implementing it in healthcare.

Evolution of Digital Twin Technology

The concept of Digital twinning dates back to the year 1970, when NASA's spacecraft Apollo 13 was onboard. The spacecraft's lunar module had alarming levels of carbon dioxide and rose to life threatening levels, the Scientists at NASA were able to communicate with the Astronauts in the spacecraft which was nearly 200,000 miles away and instructed them to utilize the materials in the spacecraft to make an air purifier. The mirrored model of the spacecraft was used by the space scientists at the ground level to assess and simulate the conditions of Apollo 13. This was the first attempt of using the DTT, however the model was analog [1, 8].

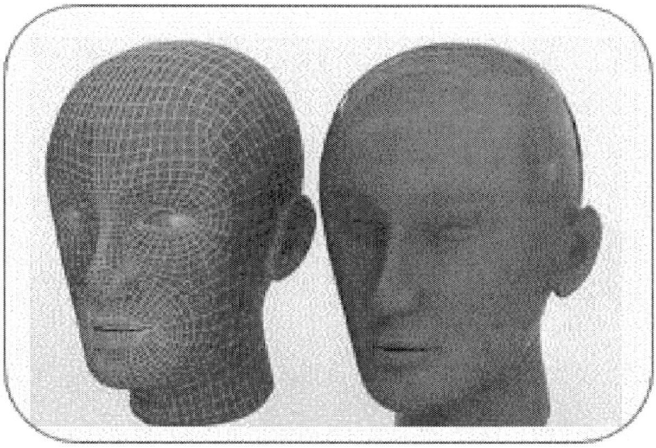

Figure 1. Digital Twin.

Later the definition and the concept of digital twin was presented by Grieves, about Product Lifecycle Management at the University of Michigan in the year 2005 [1]. Grieves defined, "Digital Twin is a virtual replica of a product that already exists or that is planned to be produced in its entirety." Although the concept evolved several decades ago, the technology spearheaded from 2017 onwards and at present it is the top strategic plans in the era of Industry 4.0.

The definition for Digital Twin has been proposed by several researchers based on their field of implementation. Hochhalter et al. [2], defines DT as a life management system for modeling and simulating the loads and environments of aerospace vehicles. Reifsnider and Majumdar [3] states that DT is useful for maintaining the onboard fleet data and health management. DT is dynamic in representing the industrial infrastructure digitally and it enables better understanding and the prediction of the performance of production machine and cost structure [4]. According to Glaessegen and Stargel, DT is an integrated multi-physic, multi scale, probabilistic simulation of a complex product and uses the best available physical models, sensor updates to mirror the life of its corresponding twin [5].

The Digital Twin represents all physical devices as they are in a real world, collects data from a real system to represent real-time information from real machinery and combines information from the real and virtual compositions. Hence, the Digital Twin can be defined as a dynamic digital model of historical and current behavior of a physical process environment helping to optimize business capability.

Definition of Digital Twin in Healthcare

DTT in healthcare is a revolution in the concept of personalized medicine. A DT has represented a virtual model of a process or product in key industries, but in healthcare it represents an individual patient.

IBM defines a DT as "the virtual representation of a physical object or system across its life-cycle." This pairing of the virtual and physical worlds allows analysis of real-time data and monitoring of responses to treatments, as well as tracking the results of behavior and lifestyle modification, to head off problems before they even occur [6].

According to Siemens, a digital twin is a four-dimensional model (here, time constitutes the 4th dimension) of a care unit, multiple departments or even an entire hospital. A digital twin links the physical and virtual worlds, turning data into actionable insights. This is a key facet of the emerging manufacturing paradigm known as Industry 4.0. [7].

Philips define digital twin as a dynamic virtual representation of a device, which is continuously fed with data from embedded sensors and software. This gives an accurate real-time status of the physical device. A model of a physical object – a 'twin' – enables you to monitor its status, diagnose issues and test solutions remotely [9].

According to Dassault systems, "The virtual twin experience of the human body will enable us to invent new ways of representing life by understanding and representing the invisible, and make a lasting contribution for the benefit of all" [10].

According to GE Healthcare, a digital twin virtualizes a hospital (or other) system to create a safe environment in which to test the impact of potential change on system performance, in other words, to play "what if?" with system dynamics [11].

Digital Twin in Healthcare Industry

The global market for digital twin in various sectors including healthcare industry are expected to have a drastic transformation from the year 2020 and expected to have the largest implementation in 2028. The reason behind this is the growth in IoT technology. By the year 2025, 89% of all IoT Platforms will contain some form of Digital Twinning capability. By 2027, Digital twinning will become standard feature/functionality for IoT Application Enablement. Above 92% of vendors already recognized the need for Industrial IoT APIs and platform integration with digital twinning functionality for industrial verticals [27, 28]. Almost 36% of industry verticals understand the benefits of digital twinning and most of them plan to incorporate within their operations by 2028. In the healthcare sector, the year 2020 is said to be the year of transformation of healthcare solutions. The digital twin technology will be the ideal blend of the doctor's imagination with the latest trends in technology. Implementation of DTs in hospitals, offers numerous benefits. It has been reported that DT could provide a 900 percent cost in savings in hospital and a 61 percent reduction in blue code hospital events [28, 29].

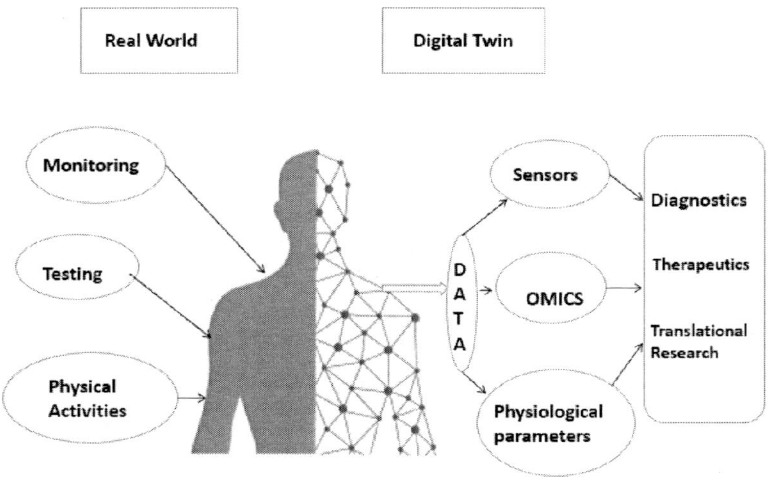

Figure 2. Digital Twin in healthcare.

Market Players in Digital Healthcare

GE Healthcare, Philips, Siemens, Alacris, IBM and Microsoft under the Azure umbrella are the front runners, with their huge databases and financial power. Dassault Systems in France branched out into health care, they had partnered with Digitwins to complete the fully functional digital twin [31].

Digital Twin Conceptual Architecture

The Digital Twin conceptual architecture provides the following steps involved in the implementation of digital twin in a more precise manner [16].

1. **Create**: The first step is to create the physical process that can measure critical inputs from the process and its surroundings (environmental data), which includes measurements from sensors

such as displacement, torque, tensile strength etc. The measurements from the sensors can be converted to secured digital information using encoders. This step is to create a process to continually update the data that is required for the analysis.

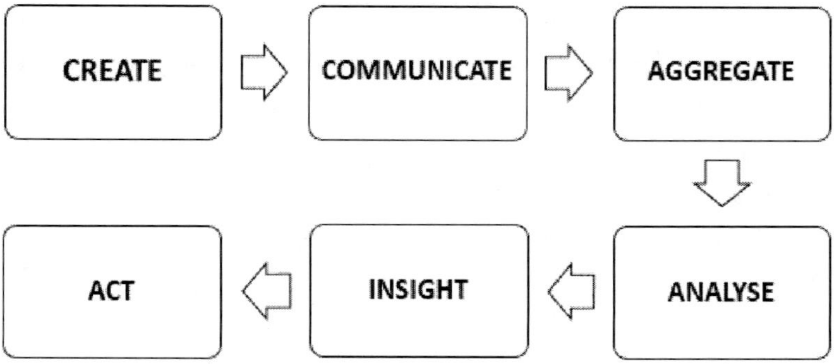

Figure 3. Key steps in Digital Twin Conceptual Architecture.

2. **Communicate**: Seamless, real-time and bidirectional integration/connectivity between the physical process and the digital platform is essential. A radical change in the digital twin technology has been made possible by the network communication. The three primary components of Industry 4.0 and the digital twin are as follows:
   a. ***Edge processing***: The edge interface connects sensors, processes signals and data from them near the source, and transfers data along to the platform. This serves to translate proprietary protocols to more easily understood data formats and reduce network communication. Major advances in this area have eliminated many bottlenecks that have limited the viability of a digital twin in the past.
   b. ***Communication interfaces***: These interfaces transfer the information from the sensor function to the integration function. The sensor can be placed almost at any location, depending on the configuration of the digital twin. The

location can be inside a factory, home, parking lot or any other location.

c. ***Edge security***: Security issues are most common and developments in the communication capabilities have created new threats and challenges. The commonly used security approaches are firewalls, application keys, encryption, and device certificates. As more and more assets become IT enabled, demand for security issues become more pressing.

3. **Aggregate**: This process supports the data collection, processing and analytics. Processing of data is done in the premises or in the cloud. The development in technology in the past few years has allowed the designers to develop scalable architectures with greater agility.
4. **Analyze**: The data is analyzed and visualized here. The advanced iterative models and analytics are utilized by the Data Scientists to gain better insights that can help in decision making.
5. **Insight**: This step gains insights from the previous step and highlights the differences between the physical world and the digital twin. The obtained insights are presented through dashboards with visualizations and indicate the areas that potentially need investigation and change.
6. **Act**: This is the final step, which closes the loop between the physical world and the digital twin. Actionable insights from the previous steps can be fed back to the physical asset and digital process to achieve the impact of the digital twin. Data from the Insights pass through decoders and are then fed into the actuators on the asset process, which are responsible for control mechanisms, or are updated in back-end systems.

The digital twin application is usually written in the primary system language of the organization, which uses the above steps to model the physical asset and processes. Standards and security measures may be applied for data management and interoperable connectivity. Enormous computing power of big data engines, analytics technologies, aggregation and integration of data along with the potential of lower cost hardware and software may lead to more realistic and sophisticated model. The conceptual architecture should be designed for flexibility and scalability in terms of analytics, processing, the number of sensors and messages, etc. These features can allow the architecture to evolve with continual and sometimes exponential changes in the market.

Development of General Digital Twin Mode for a Product

The general digital twin mode for a product consists of three entities viz. (i) physical entities in physical space (ii) virtual models in virtual space and (iii) connected data that tie the physical and virtual worlds.

I. **Physical entities**: These entities comprise of the real product that can be operated by the users. The real products are manufactured from raw materials or parts, through machining, assembly and other processes. In the course of manufacturing the physical entities, the characteristics, behaviors and performance has to be considered.

II. **Virtual models**: These are the mirror images and mapping of the physical products in the virtual space. They could reflect the whole lifecycle process, as well as simulate, monitor, diagnose, predict and control the state and behaviors of the corresponding physical entities. The virtual models include not only the geometric models, but also all rules and behaviors, such as material properties, mechanical analysis, health monitoring.

III. **Connected data:** These are the subsets of physical data and virtual data, along with some 'new data' acquired after the integration, fusion and analysis of physical data and virtual data. The parameters of the virtual models are passed to the production line and the virtual models are processed into real physical products, during the process of design and production. The product attributes, operating status and other data are fed back to the virtual models, through digital detection and measuring system to achieve a two-way data transmission process.

The Digital Twin mode is then completed by constructing the product models in the virtual space, as well as the feedback of the digital models to the physical space. Thus, the digital twin mode for a product can collect and accumulate the data continuously and help the entire lifecycle process, such as design, manufacturing, and quality inspection. These data could continue to be reused and improved, such that the digital twin mode could enable the management and tracking of the physical product with consistency.

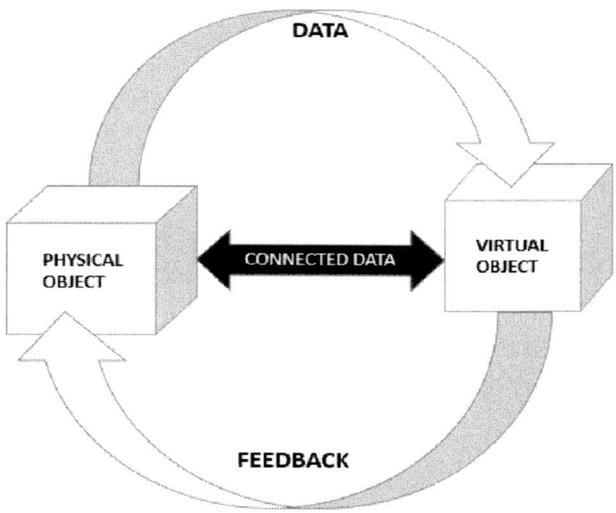

Figure 4. Process of building a functional Digital Twin.

Detailed Steps to Build the Fully Functional Digital Twin

Step 1: Creating the Virtual Model of the Physical Product

The physical product is usually designed using Computer Aided Design (CAD) and 3D modeling software. Whereas to build the virtual product, three aspects viz. elements, behaviors, and rules have to be considered [16]. The virtual product model elements include the geometric model and physical model of the product, user and environment, etc. Behavior of products and users, focus on the analysis of the product and user interaction generated by the behavior and modelling. Rules include the evaluation, optimization and forecasting models established following the law of product operation.

Step 2: Data Processing to Facilitate Decision-Making

In this process, data from the physical product and from internet are collected, integrated, analyzed and visualized. At first, data analytics is necessary to convert data into information that can be directly applied by designers for decision-making. In the second step, data collected from various sources are integrated to discover the hidden patterns that cannot be revealed based on a single data source. In the third step, data visualization technologies are incorporated to present the data with clarity. Finally, advanced artificial intelligence techniques are incorporated to improvise the Digital Twin's cognitive ability. Cognitive ability includes reasoning, problem solving and knowledge representation, which enables to make simple recommendations automatically.

Step 3: Simulate Behaviors of Physical Product in the Virtual Environment

In the past, simulation techniques employed for product design was practiced to simulate the functions of the physical product. Nowadays, Virtual Reality (VR) is used to simulate the behaviors of the physical product in the virtual world technologies are increasingly employed to support product design and virtual prototyping nowadays. VR hardware devices are readily available and can be directly adopted for digital twin.

Step 4: Sensing and Controlling the Physical Product and Virtual World

The Sensors and actuators are the two technological backbones of a digital twin. The sensors play the role in sensing the external world, whereas the actuators execute the desirable adjustments requested by DT. The Actuators adaptively controls the function, behavior and structure of the physical world. The commonly used actuators in practice are hydraulic, pneumatic, electric, and mechanical actuators [25, 26]. Augmented reality (AR) technologies can be used to reflect some parts of the virtual product back to the physical world. It enables the end users to view the real-time state of their products.

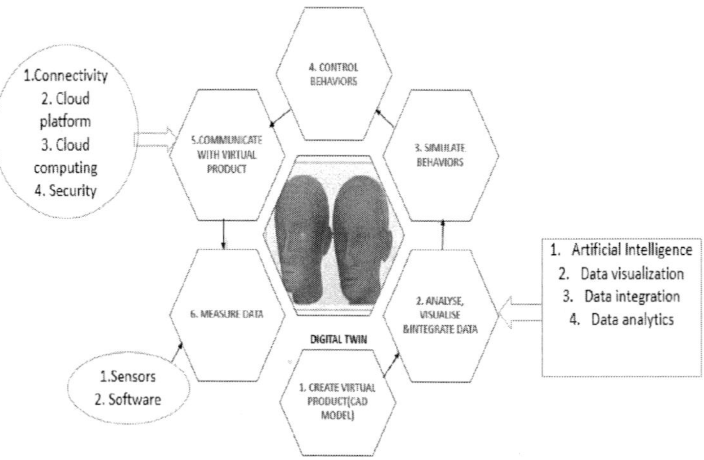

Figure 5. Development of Digital Twin – detailed flow.

Step 5: Establish Secure Connections between Physical and Virtual Product

The connections between the physical and the virtual product are established using a number of technologies, such as network communication, cloud computing and network security. Real time data is sent to the 'cloud' to power the virtual product through advanced networking technologies. The networking technologies for consumer products include, Bluetooth, QR code, barcode, Wi-Fi, Z-Wave, etc. Cloud computing technology enables the virtual product to be developed, deployed and maintained completely in the 'cloud', such that it could be accessed by both the designers and users from anywhere using Internet access. Since product data are directly and indirectly concerning user-product interactions, it is critical to guarantee the security of connections. With IoT, much effort has been taken to connect the physical and virtual product, which can be adapted for the digital twin research.

Step 6: Collect Product-Related Data

All types of product-related data that should be processed by DT has to be collected. Physical product data can be divided into product data, environmental data, customer data and interactive data. Product data consists of customer comments, viewing and download records. Interactive data consist of user-product-environment interaction, such as stress, vibration, etc. IoT and sensor technology are used to collect the above data in real time and analyze from the product manual, web page customer browsing records, download records, evaluation feedback, etc. The collected data are further fed to the Step 1, to close the loop in order to build a more functional virtual product.

Development of Healthcare-Digital Twin System

The following points will be very useful to the beginners who are venturing into healthcare digital twin system.

Developing the Digital Twin at the Organ Level

In the process of implementing the DTT in healthcare, efforts have been taken to develop the DT at the organ level. For example, the human heart can be modelled by obtaining its related parameters from the patient. The electrocardiogram results, the blood pressure readings, cardiac dynamics such as the ejection fraction, other genetic information, all these parameters necessary for assessing the function of the heart is modelled computationally [2]. The model would have the same features such as the shape, dimensions, related parameters as that of the patients' heart. The virtual model's functioning could therefore be controlled. This kind of modelling could be extended to the other organs at the level of the circulatory system or also at the pathology level, such as tumor growth, brain aneurysm, rupturing, mechanics of knee joint, etc. Artificial Intelligence is the heart of the DT system which enables the interpretation of the morphology, localization, volume and shape of the tumor [23, 24]. This kind of creating a digital twin for the organ, helps to virtually predict the reasons for the failure of the organ and also optimize the therapy.

In the current practice, electronic medical records of the patient, help to understand the conditions of the patient for robust diagnosis, in future this could be replaced by the DTs to mimic the organ by providing statistics of the patient data along with a mechanistic model to enhance the level of diagnosis and therapy [3].

Benefits to Clinicians and Patients

DTT will be a boon to both Clinicians as well as the Patients. The Clinicians need not worry whether the Patient is giving him the exact information. Also, the diagnosis can be more exhaustive and would support in decision making. The patients could experience a personalized treatment and achieve better results. Patients could get benefitted from optimized treatment planning. For example, the Digital twin could answer for whether the surgery can help the patient from cardiac resynchronization therapy.

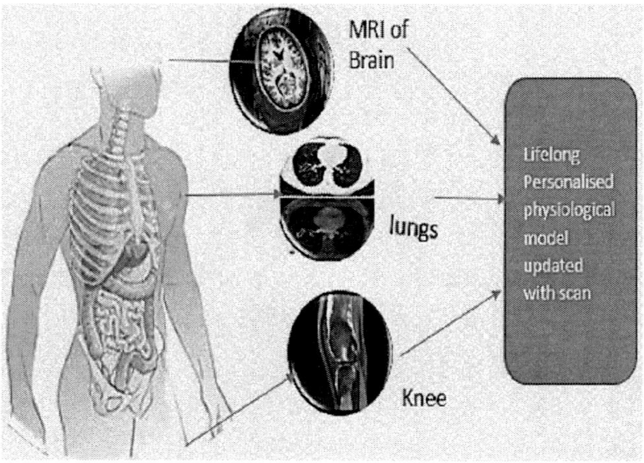

Figure 6. Personalized physiological model.

Timeframe for Clinical Practices to Adopt Digital Twin Technology

Currently the DT in healthcare is at the research level, multiple DT systems are currently in clinical testing. The time frame will depend on how far the patient can adopt with the use of this along with the clinical workflow.

Data Acquisition for Training the Digital Twin

Let us consider an example of creating the DT of the human knee, for this it is essential to obtain multiple data sets. At first, the data has to be obtained from a group of patients to train the AI model offline to build the DT. The data has to include anatomical elements of the knee and its vicinity, like the ligaments, bones, cartilage and muscles associated, along with their mechanical properties such as the stress–strain relationship and the kinetics and kinematics of the knee joint. In addition, outcome data is used to test virtual interventions or surgeries such as cartilage repair, anterior cruciate ligament reconstruction, and motion optimization. Later patient specific data has to be obtained to create the personalized model. The model hence developed will contain the generic as well as personalized information, a better inference could be made before treatment to select the best option for the patient, or during the treatment to optimize the delivery.

Source of Data to Train the AI Systems

The data required can be obtained from public databases, non-profit organizations and research organizations. The model is created with the anonymized data or the patient's own data. In case of personalized data, the patient consents the use of his/her data. The rules and regulations of the regulatory bodies has to be complied with, whatsoever the case may be. Since the data set is growing continually and becoming increasingly complex, it is suggested to use the smallest dataset, which includes the number of patients and data complexity to have a better prediction capability.

Data Privacy

The objective is having the DT for each person, such that the data could be integrated right from child birth up to a lifelong period to obtain the comprehensive physiological model, which is updated with each scan and exam. AI system will analyze and assess the data and provide suggestions for selecting the appropriate tools to make the diagnosis. The privacy of the data is of foremost concern, the collection of data has to be in strict compliance with the Data privacy law.

Application of DT

Most of the treatments include cardiac resynchronization therapy, ablation for ventricular tachycardia, tumor ablation, radiation therapy and various orthopedic procedures. The other area is "personalized health" for healthy lifestyle. Since each of us are different in our own ways, the genotype and phenotype data should also be integrated to make a complete DT.

Cost and Implementation

Artificial Intelligence powers the multiple components of DTT system, which includes model building, inference, and personalization. In healthcare, the most complex task is associated with the personalization procedure. The advancements in AI technology, improves the automation and thereby lead to cost reduction, which is optimistic in the implementation of DT in healthcare.

Recent Trends in Digital Twins for Healthcare Systems

The previous sections dealt with the processes and technology for developing a generic digital twin model. This section would throw light upon how to create digital twins for various health care applications. Medical world is looking forward to alternative medicine from physicians, without causing harm to patients but also to provide a platform for better healthcare. With emerging digital science and technology, developments in healthcare are progressing and the answer is not far away.

Hospital Ward Management Digitwin - Digital Workflow Optimization at Mater Hospital Dublin

Siemens have developed a powerful solution for intelligent decision-making in hospital system. A workflow simulation model has been developed by building a 3D computer model of any given clinical environment such as an operating room or accident and emergency. Using computing techniques, the 3D model of the system is converted into a Digital Twin via the data that was input to display everyday ward work. The operational and financial data has been given as input to simulate the actual everyday workflows. The radiology department of Mater private hospital in Dublin was redesigned using this technology. The design team redesigned the layout and architecture of the radiology department for implementing certain improvements. The design team developed a workflow simulation Digital Twin, which gave fruitful results. The wait times for CT and MRI scans were found to reduce, by an average of 19 minutes. Faster patient turnaround times were observed and a 32% increase in capacity in MRI scans and 26% in CT scans were observed. Also, the staging costs were reduced, which clearly shows that the future is in Digital Twins. It would not only help to optimize results but also to develop ward management protocol and provide cost reductions.

Electronic Medical Records - Babylon Digital Twin

Electronic Health Records or medical records are digitalized paper logs that provide a complete medical history of each individual patient. Every hospital maintains the Electronic Health Records at least for a period of two decades about what has happened to each patient. They are made accessible within the cloud-based system. Digital Twin model for Electronic Health Records would provide a visual representation of the medical history. Babylon has released its pilot Digital Twin, while still being at their initial stages. Babylon along with Bupa and other partners have teamed up to produce their "Digital Twin" in July 2018, as part of their patient health check section. Their first step is to complete a health questionnaire about past illnesses, current excise rates etc. After completion, the Digital Twin appears which is displayed as a transparent human figure, with colorful organ structures. Each of the organs and the health risk factors for future disease can be viewed by clicking on the part. Babylon uses the cutting-edge AI technology; it does this using a large database and uses a deep neural network, via deep learning technology. The data base has been created from data samples collected and inputs by their scientists and doctors, who provides up to date accurate information. The Digital twin covers up to 20 diseases which is considered as UK burden and will be expanded to 80 in the near future. With advancements in AI technology, it will not be long until they find a way to expand their numbers.

Digital Twins for Drug Development and Patient Centric Medicine

Another promising area of implementing Digital Twin is the Pharmaceutical industry. Pharma companies are developing drugs that have to be more specific and do not create any adverse reactions, to the patients. Scientists are researching completely new recovery procedures and applications that are developing technologies that can revolutionize our healthcare system. The company named AlacrisTheranostics, which is a spin-off from Max Planck Institute for Genetics, was founded in 2008. The main goal of AlacrisTheranostics is truly personalized medicine. Dr. Bodo Lange, Managing Director of the company says, "Our point is to look at how the individual patient and the particular tumor react to certain drugs," [22]. The concept of personalized medicine is administering the right medicine to individual patients. In the era of drug development, only groups of patients are addressed and not individuals were taken care off. In this way, many of the drugs do not work very effectively. Only one-third of patients responds to drug-based cancer therapies which affect the patient and is also not good for the healthcare systems. In Europe, around 200,000 people lose their lives every year due to so called adverse drug reactions. Therefore, understanding the critical information about the genes of a cancer patient would significantly reduce the number of patients who are unknowingly exposed to the side effects (and costs) of an ineffective drug. "All individuals are different," says Professor Hans Lehrach, Austrian geneticist and Emeritus Director of the Max Planck Institute for Molecular Genetics in Berlin [21]. Until now, doctors have not been able to see the molecular networks very well, and thus had a prediction problem. The only reasonable solution is to create a model for testing the digitized version of different drugs to apply the best available therapy and to exclude unwanted side effects as a prophylactic measure. In other words, to improve the quality of life and healing prospects of patients.

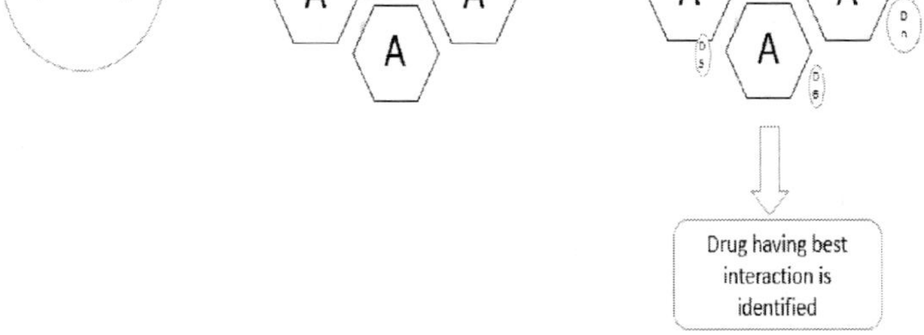

Figure 7. Digital Twin concept for personalized medicine.

The concept of digital twin for personalized medicine is illustrated in Figure 7, in which A represents the patient who has a local sign of disease. The digital twin of this patient is created in unlimited copies, using the computational models developed with disease relevant variables. Each of the twin is treated with thousands of drugs (D1, D2, ….Dn). The drug which has the best effect on the twin is found using computational studies. This drug has the best cure or it's the best digitized medicine for the twin. All other cases are ruled out. In this way, digital twin models could help to predict the drugs suitable for a specific patient, hence called personalized medicine [13]. This kind of modeling approaches can be done using the network driven models and bioinformatics tools. The protein and gene sequences are mapped using computational tools and the results obtained from the best map of protein – drug interaction will help to avoid undesirable or adverse drug reactions. The complexity of the digital twins could be increased by integrating all types of variables related to the pathogenesis.

Virtual Physiological Human (VPH)

Scientists at "The Virtual Physiological Human Institute for Integrative Biomedical Research," in Belgium are currently under the production of Virtual Physiological Human (VPH).They describe the VPH as "A world-wide community that aims to create validated in-silico models of human health and disease via the use of individualized physiology-based computer simulations in all aspects of the prevention, diagnosis, prognostic assessment, and treatment of a disease and development of a biomedical product." The three main goals of VPH are as follows: (1) the digital patient (VPH for doctors), (2) in-silico clinical trials (VPH for the biomedical and pharma industry) and (3) personal health forecasting (VPH for the patient/citizen).

Implementation of a full-fledged digital twin model is complex and there are many issues which have to be overcome [20, 21]. Human body is the most complex machine, there are numerous signaling pathways and cellular mechanisms most of which are not still fully understood. Also, disease progression and outcome are hard to validate. The database requirement is huge, an extensive database pertaining to microbiome, pharmacogenetics and tissue bank database is a must to determine all possible outcomes.

Digital Twin for Health Care Equipment Maintenance

Philips healthcare services track and analyses the technical working of MRI scanners through remote monitoring system. According to their data, an MRI scanner produces 800,000 log messages, which says how it works technically. This kind of remote monitoring system aids in solving maintenance related issues. It also helps the technician to schedule the maintenance from far and when necessary. The models developed by Philips, has not constituted a fully developed twin yet, but the underlying principle is the same. Sensors from the physical device relay the data for remote analysis. Philips have collated the technical data from more than 15,000 MRI, CT and X-ray systems from various hospitals. The data collected from the millions of data points were analyzed using machine learning techniques which lead to the identification of patterns that had significant impending issues.

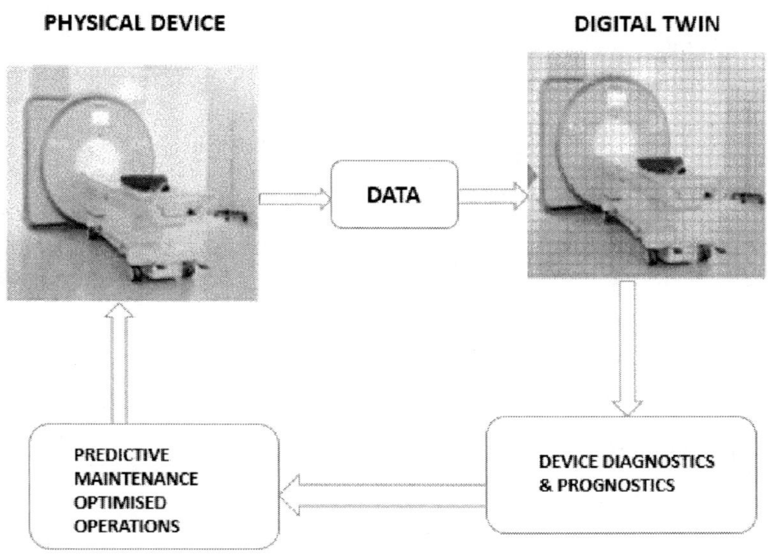

Figure 8. Digital Twin for Healthcare equipment maintenance.

Challenges and Solutions

The implementation of Digital Twin is a serious challenge in healthcare industry.

Data Handling

The challenge lies in handling the vast and enormous unstructured data. The handling of data involves data movement, storage, designing, deploying and managing algorithms for various patient types in the health care system. The computing algorithms generate even more data during the execution of the process. The data has to be completely obtained to create a fully functional twin, else the DT is incomplete and leads to the development of a faulty twin. For example, in the case of the diabetic patient, if the patient's digital twin is incomplete, the result will lead to incorrect targeting of people, therapies and resources. In case if the patient's diet is not under consideration, the algorithms for medication related decision support will not give desired results. The fault could be either because there is no way to collect this data or because the algorithm developer did not consider this parameter. A faulty twin leads to a greater number of medical errors, unnecessary expenses and unhappy patients. Therefore, while creating a digital twin, it is important to start with a genuine economic and clinical need.

Organization of Data

A well-organized data and its derivatives are essential for the computing platform to achieve a deliberate goal of relating the different "parts" of an individual to guide or automate actions for both providers and patients. In the conventional methods the blood glucose levels are being monitored continuously [12, 13]. With the advent of Digital twin platform, apart from monitoring the patients' blood glucose levels, new computing capabilities will utilize this data along with the patient's typical diet, his genetic makeup, lifestyle choices, and previous responses to different drugs to determine an appropriate response to the current blood sugar level of the patient. This process provides not only the medication management, but also gives lifestyle guidance. The challenge lies in the intelligent mapping of the patient's needs to the available resources [30, 33]. A well-organized data from the various types of patients and appropriate algorithms would provide accurate results. For instance, if a patient undergoes a surgical procedure: (a) how many days of hospital stay will be required, (b) how frequently should a patient be called to ensure he/she is sticking with a treatment regimen, (c) how often should a patient visit with his/her clinician, (d)would this patient stick to the treatment program better if he/she was given a taxi voucher to attend the therapy, (e)what drug dose is just right and (f)what is the best caloric, nutrient, or fat intake, Is a patient's weight gain indicating risk. While developing the twin, each of these questions requires different computation approaches and actuating entirely different processes. A dedicated organizational unit could be the solution to this problem for the development, monitoring and continuous improvement of the processes.

Creating Optimum Details

Creating the details required for the model poses a major challenge in creating a digital twin. The model cannot be overly simple or it could be too fast and broad, because of the complexity of acquiring and processing the data from millions of sensors and signals produced [32]. Therefore, an optimal approach which is not either too simplistic or too complex is essential to move forward.

CONCLUSION

Digital twin technology in healthcare is a data driven approach and it could improve the quality of lives in terms of medical health, sports and education. This technology makes it possible to have personalized medical care, the patients could track their health and lifestyle parameters. This concept can be applied to healthy persons, who are interested in keeping track of their health conditions. Also, the patients who use the DT can compare themselves with the database of the other patients or their previous records and modify their lifestyles accordingly. It is made possible to create digital twins of organs like the heart, or even single cells, for individual patients and run simulations in order to find out their response to different treatments.

DTT aims to reduce medical risks, improve pre-operative planning and deliver accurate therapy for patients. DTT is used in hospitals to simulate work flow processes, to identify inefficiencies and hence make improvements such as reducing patient wait time and developing strategies for efficient use of diagnostic testing equipment.

DTT plays a major role in the life cycle of product development and manufacturing processes. The concept of digital twin in healthcare has brought in new technology capabilities. The successful development of digital twins in healthcare, requires the integration of product designers, production planner and application engineers' ideas.

In future, healthcare and pharmaceutical companies may be able to start their journeys to create a digital twin with lower capital investment and shorter time to value than ever before, with enhanced patient safety. Hence creating digital twins for healthcare applications is a promising research area for integrating Artificial Intelligence, IoT and cloud-based computing platforms for solving technical, medical and ethical challenges.

REFERENCES

[1] Grieves, Michael. 2014. "*Digital twin: manufacturing excellence through virtual factory replication*." White paper 1: 1-7.

[2] Hochhalter, Jacob, William P. Leser, John A. Newman, Vipul K. Gupta, Vesselin Yamakov, Stephen R. Cornell, Scott A. Willard, and Gerd Heber. 2014. "*Coupling Damage-Sensing Particles to the Digitial Twin Concept*." NASA/TM–2014-218257. https://ntrs.nasa.gov/search.jsp?R=201400064082020-06-27T04:52:54+00:00Z.

[3] Reifsnider, Kenneth, and Prasun Majumdar. 2013. "*Multiphysics stimulated simulation digital twin methods for fleet management*," Paper presented at the 54th AIAA/ASME/ASCE/AHS/ASC Structures, Structural Dynamics, and Materials Conference, Boston, Massachusetts, April 8-11.

[4] Deloitte. 2017. "*Industry 4.0 and the Digital Twin manufacturing meets its match*." Accessed May 12. https://www2.deloitte.com/insights/us/en/focus/industry-4-0/digital-twin-technology-smart-factory.html.

[5] Glaessgen, Edward, and David Stargel. 2012. "*The digital twin paradigm for future NASA and US Air Force vehicles*." Paper presented at the 53rd AIAA/ASME/ASCE/AHS/ASC Structures, Structural Dynamics and Materials Conference 20th AIAA/ASME/AHS Adaptive Structures Conference 14th AIAA. doi: 10.2514/6.2012-1818.

[6] IBM.2019. "*Digital twin: Helping machines tell their story*," Accessed May 12. https://www.ibm.com/internet-of-things/trending/digital-twin.

[7] Siemens Healthineers. 2019. "*The value of digital twin technology, Transforming care delivery in a single department or an entire healthcare enterprise*." https://www.siemens-healthineers.com/.

[8] Fell, Jade.2017. "One giant leap for mankind [Apollo space programme]." *Engineering & Technology*. 12, no. 4, 52-53.

https://www.theguardian.com/science/2017/apr/16/apollo-13-mission-control-unsung-heroes-jim-lovell-interview.

[9] Philips. 2018. "*The rise of the Digital Twin, how healthcare can benefit*." Accessed August 30. https://www.philips.com/a-w/about/news/archive/blogs/innovation-matters/20180830-the-rise-of-the-digital-twin-how-healthcare-can-benefit.html.

[10] Dassault Systems, 2020. "*Virtual twin of the human body*," Accessed February 25. https://www.3dcadworld.com/dassault-systemes-pledges-a-virtual-twin-of-the-human-body/.

[11] GE healthcare. 2020. "*About digital Twin*." https://uscan.gehealth carepartners.com/service-about/digital-twin.

[12] Du, Jing, Qi Zhu, Yangming Shi, Qi Wang, Yingzi Lin, and Daniel Zhao. 2020." Cognition Digital Twins for Personalized Information Systems of Smart Cities: Proof of Concept." *Journal of Management in Engineering* 36, no.2: 04019052. doi: 10.1061/(ASCE)ME.1943-5479.0000740.

[13] Björnsson, Bergthor, Carl Borrebaeck, Nils Elander, Thomas Gasslander, Danuta R. Gawel, Mika Gustafsson, Rebecka Jörnsten.2020. "Digital twins to personalize medicine." *Genome Medicine* 12, no. 1: 1-4.

[14] Wagner, Raphael, Benjamin Schleich, Benjamin Haefner, Andreas Kuhnle, Sandro Wartzack, and Gisela Lanza.2019. "Challenges and Potentials of Digital Twins and Industry 4.0 in Product Design and Production for High Performance Products." *Procedia CIRP* 84: 88-93.

[15] Topol, Eric J. 2019." A decade of digital medicine innovation." *Science translational medicine* 11, no. 498: eaaw7610.

[16] Tao, Fei, Jiangfeng Cheng, Qinglin Qi, Meng Zhang, He Zhang, and Fangyuan Sui. 2018." Digital twin-driven product design, manufacturing and service with big data." *The International Journal of Advanced Manufacturing Technology* 94, no. 9-12 :3563-3576.

[17] Knapp, G. L., T. Mukherjee, J. S. Zuback, H. L. Wei, T. A. Palmer, A. De, and TarasankarDebRoy. 2017. "Building blocks for a digital twin of additive manufacturing." *Acta Materialia* 135: 390-399.

[18] Liu, Ying, Lin Zhang, Yuan Yang, Longfei Zhou, Lei Ren, Fei Wang, Rong Liu, Zhibo Pang, and M. Jamal Deen.2019. "A novel cloud-based framework for the elderly healthcare services using digital twin." *IEEE Access* 7: 49088-49101.

[19] Bruynseels, Koen, Filippo Santoni de Sio, and Jeroen van den Hoven.2018. "Digital twins in health care: ethical implications of an emerging engineering paradigm." *Frontiers in genetics* 9: 31.

[20] Lehrach, H., A. Ionescu, and N. Benhabiles.2016. "The Future of Health Care: deep data, smart sensors, virtual patients and the Internet-of-Humans." *Future health manifesto.*

[21] Lange, Klaus W., and Susanne Reichl. "Katharina M." Lange, Lara Tucha, and Oliver Tucha. 2010." The History of Attention Deficit Hyperactivity Disorder." *Attention Deficit and Hyperactivity Disorders* 2, no. 4: 241-255.

[22] Eckhart, Matthias, and Andreas Ekelhart. 2019. "Digital twins for cyber-physical systems security: State of the art and outlook." In *Security and Quality in Cyber-Physical Systems Engineering,* Springer, Cham, pp. 383-412.

[23] Grieves, Michael. 2016. "*Origins of the digital twin concept.*" Florida Institute of Technology/NASA. doi: 10.13140/RG.2.2.26367.61609.

[24] Cai, Yi, Binil Starly, Paul Cohen, and Yuan-Shin Lee. 2017. "Sensor data and information fusion to construct digital-twins virtual machine tools for cyber-physical manufacturing." *Procedia Manufacturing,* 10: 1031-1042.

[25] Qi, Qinglin, Fei Tao, Tianliang Hu, Nabil Anwer, Ang Liu, Yongli Wei, Lihui Wang, and A. Y. C. Nee. 2019. "Enabling technologies and tools for digital twin." *Journal of Manufacturing Systems,* Elsevier.

[26] Vachálek, Ján, LukásBartalský, Oliver Rovný, Dana Šišmišová, Martin Morháč, and Milan Lokšík. 2017. "*The digital twin of an industrial production line within the industry 4.0 concept.*" Presented at 21st International Conference on Process Control (PC), pp. 258-262. IEEE.

[27] The Economist. 2017. "*Millions of things will soon have digital twins*." Accessed July 13th, 2017. https://www.economist.com/business/2017/07/13/millions-of- things-will-soon-have-digital-twins.

[28] Gartner. 2017. "*Top 10 strategic technology trends for 2018*," Accessed October 4, 2017, Orlando. https://www.gartner.com/smarterwithgartner/gartner-top-10-strategic-technology-trends-for-2018/.

[29] Iscoop. 2017. "*Digital twins – rise of the digital twin in Industrial IoT and Industry 4.0*." Accesed November 2, 2017. https://www.i-scoop.eu/internet-of-things-guide/industrial-internet-things-iiot-saving-costs-innovation/digital-twins/.

[30] Neil Raden. 2020. "Digital twins for personalized medicine - a critical assessment" Accessed January 22nd, 2020. *Diginnomica*. https://diginomica.com/digital-twins-personalized-medicine-critical-assessment.

[31] Kelsey Taylor. 2019. "Digital Twin Technology benefits for healthcare" *Blog*. https://www.hitechnectar.com/blogs/digital-twin-technology-healthcare/.

[32] Don Wilcher. 2018. "The Steps in creating a digital twin." *Design News*. October 31st. https://www.designnews.com/electronics-test/steps-creating-digital-twin/34989275659708.

In: Computing Paradigms for Smart Healthcare ISBN: 978-1-53618-619-2
Editors: B. Vinoth Kumar et al.

Chapter 5

GRAPH BASED ISOTONIC SEPARATION AS A HEALTHCARE MODEL USING STATISTICAL FEATURE SELECTION

B. Malar*[*] *and R. Nadarajan
Department of Applied Mathematics and Computational Sciences,
PSG College of Technology, Coimbatore, Tamilnadu, INDIA

ABSTRACT

Recent days, breast cancer and diabetes are some of the highly prevalent diseases in the world. Efficient feature selection algorithms are required to extract important and relevant features and to construct models with high accuracy. Isotonic separation, a classification algorithm, separates data points by formulating dataset into a linear programming problem (LPP) and constructs a model from the solution of the LPP. An ideal algorithm for ordered data, it has lack of isotonic feature selection algorithms to extract isotonic features. So, this paper proposes a graph- based framework for classification called Graph-IS (Graph based Isotonic Separation) which formulates the training data as a directed acyclic graph (DAG) *G* where vertices denote the data points and

---

[*] Corresponding Author's Email: rsakthimalar@gmail.com.

arcs denotes the existence of isotonic property. This framework enables the construction of a model by mining the DAG and extracting bipartite graphs one for each class. It guarantees polynomial time to find the optimum solution of the LPP and boundary points. It also proposes a feature selection method which uses the existing notion, histograms, for extracting isotonic features from a data set. Experiments are conducted on different disease datasets and results are compared with state-of-the-art isotonic separation techniques. Results reveal that histogram-based feature selection not only selects isotonic features but also improves the performance of graph based isotonic separation with its counterparts.

Keywords: directed acyclic graph (DAG), Graph-IS

INTRODUCTION

In the contemporary era, many diseases are highly prevalent in the world. Some of the life-threatening diseases are breast cancer, heart attack and diabetes. For example, 1 in 22 women are predicted to develop the disease breast cancer which is one of the deadliest diseases in India. The five-year survival rate of this disease among Indian women is about 60%. As per WHO's latest assessment, cancer cases in India will multiply five times over the next decade (by 2025) with more women falling prey to it than men. The data collected from www.breastcancerindia.com web site, shows that one fourth of all female cancer cases are breast cancers. In India, over 10 lakh new cases of cancer are diagnosed every year. However, due to late diagnosis, over 7 lakh people die from the disease each year. Projections by Indian Council of Medical Research show that India is likely to have over 17.3 lakh new cases of cancer and over 8.8 lakh deaths due to disease by 2020. So, a decision support system is required to predict whether given tumor is malignant or benign. Machine learning algorithms play a vital role in diagnosis of diseases using abundant historical data.

Isotonic separation [2] is one of the machine learning algorithms to separate d-dimensional data in a domain where an isotonic property exists. In lecturer evaluation, for instance, the isotonic consistency condition can be formed by stating that a faculty with higher credits (punctuality, teaching, evaluation, etc.) is most likely to be better than those with lower credits. Such isotonic consistency conditions are prevalent not only in healthcare domain such as breast cancer diagnosis [22] and cancer prognosis [22] but also in other applications including internet content filtering [12] firm bankruptcy prediction [21].

Given a historical training data with n data points and d features/dimensions in a binary classification problem, the rationale behind isotonic separation is to formulate a maximum flow network with n+2 vertices and m+2n edges where $n \leq m \leq \frac{n(n-1)}{2}$ for constructing a model and classifying unknown test data [1]. The dual of maximum flow network can also be deployed as a linear programming problem (LPP) with n variables and m constraints [5] [19]. The isotonic consistency condition requires a quasi-order on the set of data points, which becomes the constraints of maximum flow network model or linear programming (LP) model. Based on the solution obtained from any one of the above models, the d-dimensional input space is partitioned into isotonic region1 for each class and a non-isotonic region 2. The unknown test data will be classified based on the region where it appears in the input space. Thus, the performance of isotonic separation depends to a great extent on the number of training instances n, the number of constraints m, the dimensionality d and the time complexity to solve the LP or network model.

One of the key challenges in isotonic separation is extraction of isotonic features from given set of features. Besides feature selection metrics such as entropy, information gain, many computational techniques are also available in literature [8] [9].

To address the extraction of isotonic features, this paper proposes a new framework for isotonic separation called graph based isotonic separation (GRAPH-IS). This framework models the LPP as a directed acyclic graph *G*, deploys a newly proposed algorithm to construct a model by mining the graph and extracts boundary points from the solution of the

---

[1] A region where data points satisfy isotonic consistency condition.

[2] A region where isotonic consistency condition does not exist.

LPP. It also uses histogram to select isotonic features in a data set. Experiments are conducted on diverse disease datasets to validate the results.

The remaining part of the paper is structured as follows: Section 2 presents the preliminaries associated with graph theory and isotonic separation. Section 3 gives the graph-based model for isotonic separation. Section 4 demonstrates the proposed work with a case study. Section 5 presents the experimental and time complexity analysis of Graph-IS and comparative study with other state of the art algorithms. Section 6 presents concluding remarks.

BACKGROUND

This section presents the definitions and terminologies related to graph theory and isotonic separation [24] [2]

Definition 1: A directed graph $G = (V, E)$ contains a vertex set V and an edge set E. A weighted digraph G is a 5-tuple, $G = \langle V, E, W \rangle$ where V be a set of vertices, E be a set of edges and W be a set of weights assigned to V. Edge (i, j) originates at vertex i and terminates at vertex j.

Definition 2: Directed Acyclic Graph (DAG) is a directed graph with no cycles.

Definition 3: A graph G is bipartite if its set of vertices can be partitioned into two non-empty subsets X and Y so that there is no arc uv of G with u and v both in X or both in Y.

Isotonic Separation

Let **T** be a dataset with n instances in which each instance $\mathbf{x}_i = (x_{i1}, x_{i2}, ..., x_{id})$ is a data point in the d-dimensional feature space and has a class label $y_i \in \{0,1\}$. The set of instances in **T** is partitioned into two disjoint classes T_0 and T_1, where $T = T_0 \cup T_1$.

$$T_0 = \{(\boldsymbol{x}_i, y_i) | y_i = 0\}$$
$$T_1 = \{(\boldsymbol{x}_i, y_i) | y_i = 1\} \tag{1}$$

The basic assumption in the isotonic separation [2] is an isotonic consistency condition between objects and it results a quasi-ordering relation *R* as in Equation (2).

$$R = \{(i, j) | \ \mathbf{x}_i \succ \mathbf{x}_j\} \tag{2}$$

The key objective of isotonic separation is to obtain an isotonic function $\hat{f}: X \rightarrow \{0,1\}$ which maps any data point in the d-dimensional real space into class labels accurately. Isotonic function is a non increasing function $\hat{f}$ on **T** to {0, 1} that is isotonic with respect to R with minimum misclassifications. A penalty ω_i is assigned to each instance using the following rule:

$$\omega_i = \begin{cases} \alpha & f(\mathbf{x}_i) = 1 \text{ and } \hat{f}(\mathbf{x}_i) = 0 \\ \beta & f(\mathbf{x}_i) = 0 \text{ and } \hat{f}(\mathbf{x}_i) = 1 \\ 0 & f(\mathbf{x}_i) = \hat{f}(\mathbf{x}_i) \end{cases} \tag{3}$$

Isotonic function is obtained by modeling the LPP with an objective of minimizing the total misclassification penalty. The solution to the LPP is used to find the classification model. The LPP is formulated as follows:

min

$$\alpha \sum_{\mathbf{x}_i \in \mathbf{T}_1} (1 - y_i) + \beta \sum_{\mathbf{x}_i \in \mathbf{T}_0} y_i$$

subject to the constraints (4)

$$y_i - y_j \geq 0 \; for \; (i, j) \in R$$

$$0 \leq y_i \leq 1 \; for \; \mathbf{x}_i \in \mathbf{T}$$

Here y_i is a binary variable and it can be a real variable in [0, 1]. In the objective function of Eqn. (4), $\sum_{X_i \in T_1}(1 - y_i)$ and $\sum_{Xi \in T_0} y_i$denote the number of type-1 and type-2 errors respectively. Let $\mathbf{Y}^*$ be the optimum or near optimum solution of the LPP and it is isotonic with respect to *R*. Boundary points for each class are obtained using the equation given below and these points are used to classify the unknown test instance.

$$\mathbf{T}_1^* = \{\mathbf{x}_i \mid y_i^* = 1 \text{ and } \nexists y_j^* \in \mathbf{Y}^*, i \neq j, \; y_j^* = 1 \text{ and } (i, j) \in R\}$$
$$\mathbf{T}_0^* = \{\mathbf{x}_i \mid y_i^* = 0 \text{ and } \nexists y_j^* \in \mathbf{Y}^*, i \neq j, \; y_j^* = 0 \text{ and } (j, i) \in R\} \quad (5)$$

where $\mathbf{T}_1^* \neq \phi$ and $\mathbf{T}_0^* \neq \phi$. The *d*-dimensional space is separated into three regions based on boundary points:

$$Z_0 = \{\mathbf{x}_j \mid \; (i, j) \in R \text{ where } y_i^* = 0\}$$
$$Z_1 = \{\mathbf{x}_j \mid (j, i) \in R \text{ where } y_i^* = 1\} \quad (6)$$
$$Z_2 = \Re^d - (Z_0 \cup Z_1)$$

In the test set, for every instance $\mathbf{x}_h$, whose feature vector is $(x_{h1}, x_{h2}, \ldots, x_{hd})$, classification is done as follows: If $\mathbf{x}_h$ lies in the area of Z_1, then $\mathbf{x}_h$ belongs to class $\mathbf{T}_1$. If $\mathbf{x}_h$ lies in the area of Z_0, then $\mathbf{x}_h$ belongs to class $\mathbf{T}_0$.

$$y_h^* = \begin{cases} 1 & \text{if } \mathbf{x}_h \text{ lies in } Z_1 \\ 0 & \text{if } \mathbf{x}_h \text{ lies in } Z_0 \end{cases} \tag{7}$$

If $\mathbf{x}_h$ lies in Z_2, where none of the instances exist and isotonic consistency condition cannot be able to determine its class label. In this scenario, the distance between the unknown object $\mathbf{x}_h$ and undominated points are measured. The object $\mathbf{x}_h$ is assigned to the class with minimum distance.

$$\begin{aligned} D_{h1} &= \beta \min\left\{ \sum_{k=1}^{d} \max(x_{hk} - x_{ik}, 0)\ \mathbf{x}_i \in Z_1 \right\} \\ D_{h0} &= \alpha \min\left\{ \sum_{k=1}^{d} \max(x_{ik} - x_{hk}, 0)\ \mathbf{x}_i \in Z_0 \right\} \\ y_h^* &= \begin{cases} 1 & D_{h1} < D_{h0} \\ 0 & \text{otherwise} \end{cases} \end{aligned} \tag{8}$$

Variants of Isotonic Separation

Isotonic Separation is a data classification technique which has been proposed for two category separation and generalized to multi category separation [2]. The key issues identified in isotonic separation were feature selection and problem size reduction. Problem size reduction focuses on reducing the number of constraints or decision variables in the LPP. Authors reduced the problem size by removing reflexive and transitively implied constraints from the relation *R*.

Soft set based isotonic separation (SOFIA-IS) is proposed to address the issue of problem size reduction in the LPP [16]. This approach selects the relevant and important instances using a new instance selection algorithm called SOFIA. SOFIA uses soft set with statistical parameters for obtaining the condensed dataset. This reduced dataset is used as the training set for isotonic separation. But the limitation of this approach is that it is applicable only for spherical data sets due to the selection of statistical parameters.

For firm bankruptcy prediction, the isotonic separation method was applied on a set of 23 financial ratios as features [21]. To filter unwanted internet content, isotonic separation was deployed using the platform for internet content selection (PICS) rating scheme [12]. A new approach has been proposed to refine the boundary points. This approach compares the test data with the training set for isotonicity and boundary points are updated. The limitation of this approach is that it is computationally expensive and it consumes more memory and resources due to the availability of training data at the time of testing.

An improved version of isotonic separation was proposed by Ryu et al. to reduce the number of constraints and decision variables in the LPP. This scheme allows finding a maximal subset of data points for each class. As a result, the decision variables and constraints are reduced substantially. This method was trained and tested with 699 points which resulted in higher accuracy.

Evolutionary isotonic separation (EIS) has been proposed to address the issue of solving large scale LPP in isotonic separation [15]. This approach uses genetic algorithm [6] [8] [9] to find the optimum or near optimum solution for the LPP. A slack vector is introduced for obtaining the feasible solution. The shortcoming of this approach is that the convergence criterion is not deterministic and this method is expensive for large datasets to converge.

A PSO (Particle Swarm Optimization) based isotonic separation has been proposed to address the concerns in EIS [17]. This scheme has introduced a new deterministic convergence criterion which measures the number of data points that violates the isotonic property. It makes an algorithm to terminate with minimum number of misclassifications. Albeit this algorithm takes less time for even large data sets when compared with EIS, it has a limitation that this approximates the solution for the LPP.

Feature selection focuses on selecting relevant features to construct the model. Authors adopted backward sequential elimination method [22] [11] to select relevant features in the dataset. This motivates us to propose a new statistical method to select the best isotonic features from the given data and propose a graph-based method to extract the model and boundary points in isotonic separation.

Problem Statement

Graph-IS, per se unique model in isotonic separation, extracts isotonic features using histogram, formulates the LPP as a graph, proposes a method to construct a model from a graph.

Graph Based Isotonic Separation

A graph-based framework for isotonic separation, GRAPH-IS, comprises of four phases. First, isotonic features are extracted using a histogram-based method and a data set with isotonic features is portrayed as a DAG. Then it finds an optimum or near optimum solution using simplex method. Finally, it constructs a model by mining the DAG and extracts the bipartite graph.

Histogram-Based Feature Selection

The histogram-based feature selection technique works in two stages. In the first stage, the data set is split into partitions based on the values of class variable. Then histogram is drawn class-wise for each feature and isotonic features are identified from histograms.

The data points in *D* fall into one of two disjoint classes A_0 and A_1 based on their output labels.

$$A_1 = \{\mathbf{x}_i \mid \mathbf{x}_i \in D \text{ and } y_i = 1\}$$
$$A_0 = \{\mathbf{x}_i \mid \mathbf{x}_i \in D \text{ and } y_i = 0\} \quad (9)$$

Each partition is visualized with respect to individual features using histogram (Han 2005) which are then analysed for the existence of isotonic property.

Let X be a feature which takes k ordered values $(v1, v2, ..., vK)$ and its probability distribution $(p_{v1}^0, p_{v2}^0, ..., p_{vK}^0)$ for class A0 and $(p_{v1}^1, p_{v2}^1, ..., p_{vK}^1)$ for class A1. A feature X is said to be isotonic if the frequency of smaller values of a feature is high in one class and the frequency of bigger values of a feature is low in another class.

Based on the above definition, isotonic features are identified and included in the feature subset. Let $(d_{v1}, d_{v2}, ..., d_{vK})$ be the difference between class wise probability of ordered values $(v1, v2, ..., vK)$ and is calculated as follows:

$$d_k = p_k^1 - p_k^0 \text{ for } v1 \le k \le vK \quad (10)$$

Isotonic property is measured based on this difference d_k. A feature is said to be perfectly isotonic, if d_k is growing from negative to positive or reducing from positive to negative. It can be defined as follows:

$$feature = \{isotonic \text{ if } d_{v1} \le d_{v2} \le ... \le d_{vk} \quad (11)$$

If a feature is not perfectly isotonic, then the occurrence of violation in d is calculated and a feature with minimum number of violations is chosen.

Graph Formulation

Let G = (V, E) be a directed graph with a vertex set V and an edge set E. Each vertex in G denotes a data point in A and forms a vertex set $V = \{v_i \mid \mathbf{x}_i \in A\}_{i=1}^{n}$. Each vertex v_i is associated with set of feature values of a corresponding data point, an actual class label y_i and a predicted class label $\hat{y}_i$. It can be represented as a triplet $\langle \mathbf{x}, y, \hat{y} \rangle$ where

$$y = \{y_i \mid v_i \in V \text{ and } y_i \in \{0,1\}\}_{i=1}^{n} \tag{12}$$

$$\hat{y} = \{\hat{y}_i \mid v_i \in V \text{ and } \hat{y}_i \in \{0,1\}\}_{i=1}^{n} \tag{13}$$

The edge set E denotes a set of edges and each denotes an isotonic consistency condition between vertices v_i and v_j. Edge set is defined as follows.

$$E = \{(v_i, v_j) \mid v_i, v_j \in V \text{ and } x_{ik} \geq x_{jk} \;\; \forall k \;\; 1 \leq k \leq d\} \tag{14}$$

From the graph G, transitively implied edges are removed in order to minimize the number of edges. Now G can be considered as a directed acyclic graph (DAG) and an LPP. The optimum solution for the LPP can be obtained using any of the linear programming techniques.

Isotonic Separator

After finding an optimum solution for the LPP, the next step is to construct an isotonic separator for each class. Isotonic separator is a set of boundary points for each class. Let $\hat{\mathbf{y}} = \{\hat{y}_j\}_{j=1}^{n}$ be the optimum solution of the LPP and it is obtained from the constrained BFS approach. Boundary points are obtained by extracting a bipartite graph for each class from the given graph G.

Let $G_0 =< V_{00}V_{01} >$ and $G_1 =< V_{10}V_{11} >$ are two bipartite graphs in G. Let V_{00} and V_{01} are the partitions for G_0 and V_{10} and V_{11} are the partitions for G_1. Vertex $v_i \in V_{11}$ iff,

1. $\hat{y}_i = 1$
2. For all adjacent edges v_j associated with v_i, $(v_i, v_j) \in E$, $\hat{y}_j = 0$.

Then, the vertices v_j are included in V_{10}. Similarly, Vertex $v_i \in V_{00}$ iff,

1. $\hat{y}_i = 0$
2. For all incident edges v_j associated with v_i, $(v_j, v_i) \in E$, $\hat{y}_j = 1$.

The vertices v_j are included in V_{01}. Let E_1 be the edge set which connects vertices of two partitions V_{10} and V_{11} in G_1 and E_0 be the edge set which connects vertices of two partitions V_{00} and V_{01} in G_0.

$$
\begin{aligned}
&V_{11} = \{v_i \mid \hat{y}_i = 1 \text{ and } \nexists v_j \in V, i \neq j, \hat{y}_j = 1 \text{ and } (v_i, v_j) \in E\} \\
&V_{10} = \{v_j \mid v_i \in V_{11}, \hat{y}_i = 1 \text{ and } v_j \in V, i \neq j, \hat{y}_j = 0 \text{ and } (v_i, v_j) \in E\} \\
&E_1 = \{(v_i, v_j) \mid v_i \in V_{11}, v_j \in V_{10} \text{ and } (v_i, v_j) \in E\} \\
&G_1 = \langle V_1, E_1 \rangle \text{ where } V_1 = V_{10} \cup V_{11} \\
&V_{00} = \{v_i \mid \hat{y}_i = 0 \text{ and } \nexists v_j \in V, i \neq j, \hat{y}_j = 0 \text{ and } (v_j, v_i) \in E\} \\
&V_{01} = \{v_j \mid v_i \in V_{00}, \hat{y}_i = 0 \text{ and } v_j \in V, i \neq j, \hat{y}_j = 1 \text{ and } (v_j, v_i) \in E\} \\
&E_0 = \{(v_i, v_j) \mid v_i \in V_{00}, v_j \in V_{01} \text{ and } (v_i, v_j) \in E\} \\
&G_0 = \langle V_0, E_0 \rangle \text{ where } V_0 = V_{00} \cup V_{01}
\end{aligned}
\tag{15}
$$

From the bipartite graphs G_0 and G_1, boundary points for each class are obtained as follows:

$$B_0 = \{v_i \mid v_i \in V_0 \text{ and } \hat{y}_i = 0\}$$
$$B_1 = \{v_i \mid v_i \in V_1 \text{ and } \hat{y}_i = 1\} \tag{16}$$

Test data is classified using equation (8).

Theoretical Analysis

This section analyses the time complexity of the proposed graph based isotonic separation with histogram-based feature selection technique.

Lemma 1: In graph G, $|v| = n$ and $|E| = O(n^2)$

Proof

Since each instance in the data set is represented as a vertex, $|v| = n$. Each ordered pair (i, j) in R is a directed edge from v_i to v_j in G. The number of ordered pairs in R is in the range of $n \le |R| \le \frac{n(n-1)}{2}$. So $|E| = O(n^2)$.

Lemma 2: The graph G is a directed acyclic graph (DAG).

Proof

From lemma 1, it is proved that the graph G is a directed graph. To prove that G is acyclic, the relation $R = \{(i, j) \mid \mathbf{x}_i \ge \mathbf{x}_j\}$ is used. Since R is assumed to be a quasi (reflexive and transitive) relation, R does not have reflexive pairs and there is no self-loop in G. Since R is not symmetric, there is no cycle between v_i and v_j. Since R is assumed as a transitive relation, that is for all edges (v_i, v_j), if $(v_i, v_j) \in E$ and $(v_j, v_k) \in E$, then $(v_i, v_k) \notin E$, so there is no cycle between the vertices v_i and v_k through v_j. Hence the graph G is proved as a DAG.

Lemma 3: The time complexity of Graph-IS is $O(\max(n^2 d, n^3))$ which is equivalent to $O(n^3)$.

Proof

Given a training set with n instances in a d-dimensional data space, the time complexity of histogram-based feature selection algorithm is O(nd). The time complexity to check isotonic consistency constraints is $O(n^2 d)$.The time to formulate the LPP using graph data structure is $\theta(n^2)$. The time complexity to find out and eliminate transitive pairs is $\theta(n^3)$. Let m be the number of constraints (edges) and n be the number of decision variables (vertices) in the LPP (graph). The time complexity of finding a solution to the LPP is $O(n^3)$. The time complexity to extract a bipartite graph is $O(n^2)$. So, the time complexity of Graph-IS is $O(\max(n^2 d, n^3))$ which is equivalent to $O(n^3)$.

CASE STUDY

The main objective of Graph-IS is to construct an efficient classifier using the training set presented in Table 1. The training set includes instance number, nine features named as F1 to F9, and a class label (1 – malignant 0 – benign). As a result of the isotonic consistency condition, relation R is obtained. After eliminating reflexive and transitive pairs from

R, the resulting relation is transformed into a graph G as shown in Figure 1. Each instance is represented as a vertex and every ordered pair (i, j) in R creates an arc from i to j. Simplex technique is applied to find the optimum solution for the LPP.

From the optimum solution, graph is mined and two bipartite graphs (G1, G0) are extracted as shown in Figure 2. Boundary points are obtained as follows: the vertices that are in V11 = {1, 2, 6, 9, 10, 11, 13, 14} for class 1 and the vertices that are in V00 = {3,4} for class 0. These boundary points are used for classifying unknown instances in the test set.

Table 1. Sample dataset

ins_no	F_1	F_2	F_3	F_4	F_5	F_6	F_7	F_8	F_9	*Y*
1	10	10	10	10	10	1	8	8	8	1
2	5	3	4	1	8	10	4	9	1	1
3	1	3	1	2	2	2	5	3	2	0
4	3	3	2	1	2	3	3	1	1	0
5	10	10	10	2	10	10	5	3	3	1
6	5	3	5	1	8	10	5	3	1	1
7	1	1	1	2	2	1	3	1	1	0
8	1	1	1	1	2	1	2	1	1	0
9	5	3	3	3	6	10	3	1	1	1
10	5	8	8	8	5	10	7	3	1	1
11	4	4	4	4	6	5	7	3	1	1
12	3	1	1	1	2	0	3	1	1	0
13	10	8	8	2	8	10	4	8	10	1
14	9	8	8	5	6	2	4	10	4	1

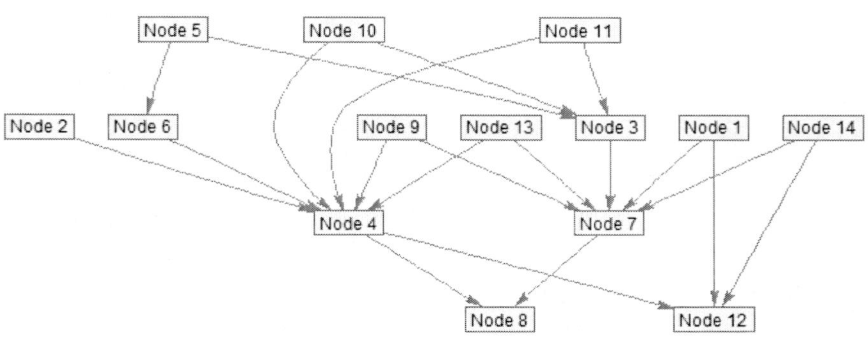

Figure 1. Graph model of the LPP for the sample dataset in Table 1.

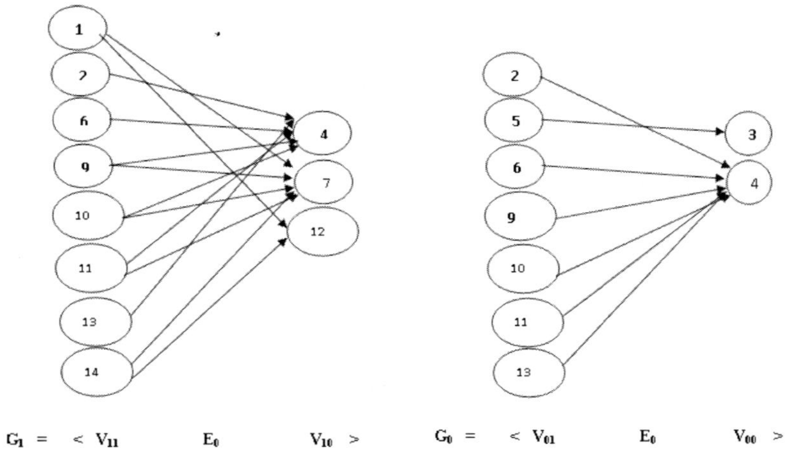

Figure 2. Bipartite graphs as a result of mining boundary points

EXPERIMENTAL ANALYSIS

To assess the computational performance of the proposed graph framework and histogram-based feature selection technique, experiments are conducted on diverse data sets and results are reported.

Experimental Setup

The pre-requisites for isotonic separation are that the existence of isotonic property in the datasets and the class labels are binary and very few data sets possess these prerequisites. Table 2 lists these data sets [18] and their properties such as # data points and features.

Experiments are conducted using hold out method which splits data set in to training and test set in the ratio of 2:1. The proposed histogram-based feature selection is performed on all the data sets and features are selected. Experiments are conducted using variants of isotonic separation with all and reduced features. Other characteristics such as number of decision variables, constraints, F-measure and training time are reported.

Table 2. Data sets

Dataset	Size (n)	Features (d)
Haberman Survival (HS)	306	3
Wisconsin Breast Cancer Dataset (WBCD)	699	9
Pima Indians (PI)	768	8

Experimental Results

This paper has a couple of significant contributions: (i) a histogram-based feature selection algorithm for extracting isotonic features (ii) Graph based model of isotonic separation with a new labeling technique for labeling vertices in a graph. Therefore, experiments are conducted on data sets so as to prove the significance of contributions by comparing results with other state of the art isotonic separation algorithms and machine learning algorithms.

Analysis of Histogram Based Feature Selection

The histogram for Haberman survival dataset which has the survival report of patients who had undergone surgery for breast cancer is reported in Figure 3. It reveals that the features, age of patient and number of auxiliary nodes, are isotonic because it is inferred from histogram that younger patients are more probable to survive than older patients and patients with less number auxiliary nodes are more likely to survive than those with many nodes.

Figure 4 reports the histogram for Pima Indians diabetes data set which includes the details of female patients with at least 21 years old of Pima Indian heritage. The features number of times pregnant, serum insulin, BMI, pedigree function and age are isotonic and selected for classification.

Figure 5 reports the histogram for Wisconsin Breast cancer data set. All features are monotonic and included in the feature subset.

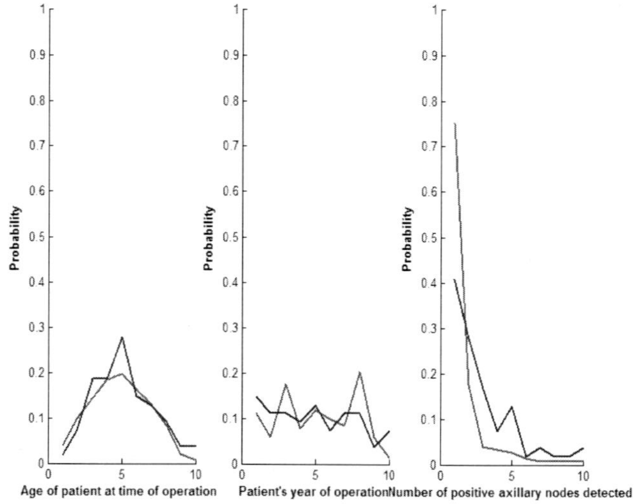

* Blue curve: patients died within five years
Red curve: patients survive for five years or longer

Figure 3. Histogram Plot for Haberman Survival data set.

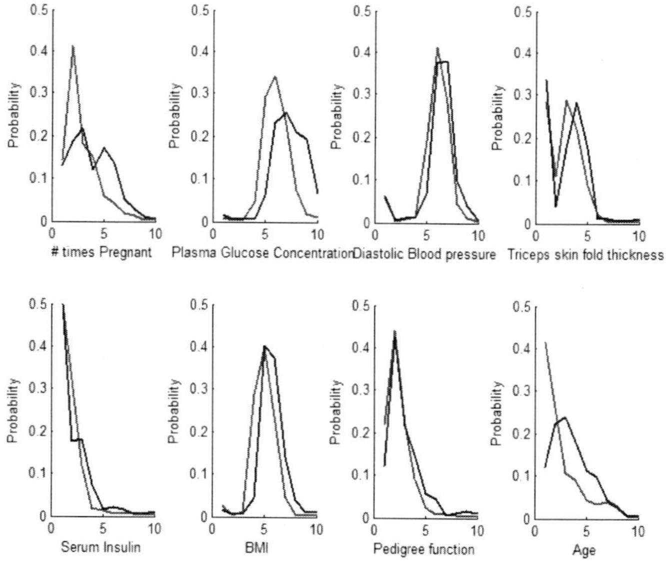

* Blue: class with diabetic patients Red: class with non diabetic patients

Figure 4. Histogram plot for Pima Indians Diabetes Dataset.

Table 3 shows the classification performance of state-of-the-art isotonic separation algorithms with and without histogram-based feature selection on the above data sets. Results reveal that the variants of isotonic separation with feature selection perform better than those without feature selection on small, medium and large data sets.

Table 4 shows the impact of feature selection in size of the LPP on the above-mentioned data sets. Generally, size of LPP is determined by number of constraints and decision variables in an LPP. Results show that number of constraints in the LPP is increased as features are reduced. It infers that histogram-based feature selection increases monotonicity in the data set as it chooses isotonic features. As a consequence, number of ordered pairs and in turn constraints have also been increased. However, most of the variants of isotonic separation except IS (isotonic separation) are capable of solving LPP with many decision variables and constraints and produce better model and significant results. It is obvious from the results that histogram-based feature selection improves the classification performance of isotonic classifiers.

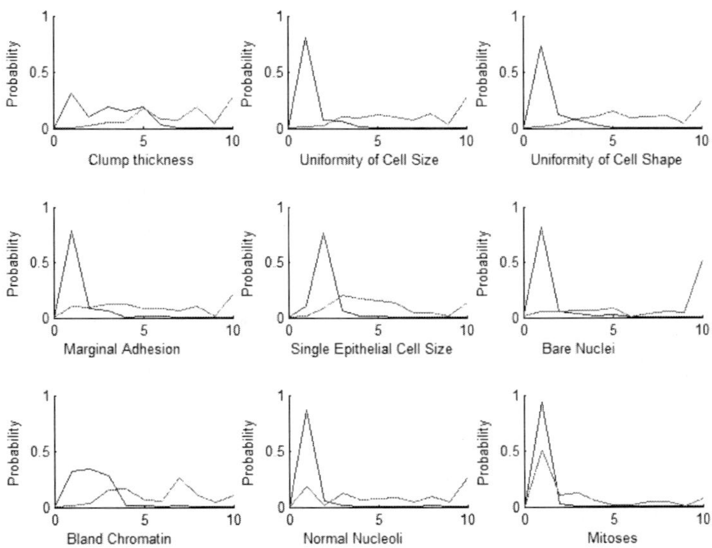

* Blue: class with benign patients Red: class with malignant patients

Figure 5. Histogram Plot for WBCD.data set

Table 3. Comparative study of F-measure between isotonic separation and its variants on different data sets

Dataset	Haberman Survival	WBCD	Pima Indians
IS	97.4	97.5	96.1
IS with FS	98.5	99.1	96.8
EIS	96.8	97.2	95.2
EIS with FS	97.0	98.4	95.7
MeHeIS-CPSO	97.2	97.4	95.8
MeHeIS-CPSO with FS	98.0	99.0	96.2
SOFIA-IS	98.2	98.0	96.0
SOFIA-IS with FS	98.3	99.2	96.5
Graph-IS	97.6	97.4	95.8
Graph-IS with FS	98.5	99.3	96.7

Table 4. Size of the LPP on different data sets before and after histogram-based feature selection

Dataset	Decision Variables (n)		Constraints (m)	
	Before Feature Selection	After Feature Selection	Before Feature Selection	After Feature Selection
Haberman Survival	200	200	574	890
WBCD	460	460	6899	7213
Pima Indians	500	500	3286	3858

Analysis of Graph-IS

In order to assess the performance of Graph-IS, experiments are conducted on datasets and results are reported. The training set is transformed into a directed acyclic graph G which comprises of 630 nodes and 2932 edges on average and vertices of G are labeled using simplex method. The solution vector is taken and considered for constructing isotonic separator. The average boundary points for malignant and benign class are 46 and 68 respectively. Then, mean and 95% confidence interval on the mean for the measures (accuracy, precision, recall, F-measure and FPR) [3] [7] [10] [13] [14] [20] [23] of 10-trials are calculated and reported in Table 5. Results reveal that Graph-IS gives better results than state of the art isotonic separation algorithms and other machine learning algorithms. This has occurred because misclassifications in the optimum solution of the LPP obtained from the Graph-IS are less than other frameworks.

Table 5. 95% confidence interval for the mean of Accuracy, Precision, Recall, False positive rate and F-measure values of Graph-IS and other machine learning techniques on WBCD

Algorithms	Accuracy (%)	Precision (%)	Recall (%)	FPR (%)	F-measure (%)
C4.5	92.4 ± 3.9	93.4 ± 3.0	93.0 ± 3.2	8.2 ± 4.6	92.9 ± 3.4
SVM	96.6 ± 2.0	96.8 ± 2.0	96.5 ± 2.3	3.4 ± 2.0	96.5 ± 2.3
IS	97.5 ± 0.8	96.1 ± 2.5	95.4 ± 2.7	2.7 ± 2.7	95.6 ± 3.1
EIS	97.1 ± 1.7	92.6 ± 3.4	98.8 ± 2.7	2.6 ± 1.8	96.9 ± 3.9
SOFIA-IS	97.2 ± 0.8	94.0 ± 3.9	99.5 ± 1.6	4.4 ± 2.9	96.6 ± 2.4
MeHeIS-CPSO	98.2 ± 1.1	97.0 ± 1.3	98.5 ± 0.7	1.0 ± 0.3	97.3 ± 1.2
Graph-IS	**98.6 ± 1.1**	**97.5 ± 1.8**	**98.4 ± 0.9**	**1.0 ± 0.2**	**97.6 ± 2.1**

Table 6 portrays the comparative study of all the state-of-the-art isotonic separation algorithms on different data sets that satisfy isotonic properties using accuracy, precision, recall, FPR and f-measure. It is inferred from the results that the proposed graph-is method provides significant results in 80% of the cases.

Table 6. Comparative Study of Accuracy, Precision, Recall, FPR and F-measure in IS, EIS, MeHeIS-CPSO and Graph-IS

Datasets	Algorithms	Accuracy (%)	Precision (%)	Recall (%)	FPR (%)	F-measure (%)
Haberman	MeHeIS-CPSO	98.2	97.0	98.5	1.0	97.7
	EIS	96.5	95.7	98.2	2.8	96.9
	IS	97.6	97.5	98.3	3.1	97.6
	Graph-IS	99.3	98	98.3	1.9	98.1
Pima Indians	MeHeIS-CPSO	98.7	97.5	98.5	3.0	97.6
	EIS	97.7	97.6	97.8	2.6	97.7
	IS	97.9	98.0	98.1	2.0	98.0
	Graph-IS	99	98.6	99.7	1.3	99.1
WBCD	MeHeIS-CPSO	98.9	97.5	99.5	1.9	97.8
	EIS	97.2	96.3	98.0	3.0	97.6
	IS	98.0	97.5	98.3	3.0	97.6
	Graph-IS	98.6	97.5	98.3	1.5	97.9

Table 7. Comparison of time complexities of isotonic separation and its variants

Algorithm		Time Complexity	
Classification	**For solving LPP**	**For solving LPP**	**Classification**
Isotonic separation	Simplex method	$O((m+n)m^2)$	$O(n^3+(m+n)m^2)$
EIS	Evolutionary Framework	$O(Np(m+n))$	$O(\max(Np(m+n), n^3))$
MeHeIS-CPSO	PSO	$O(Np(m+n))$	$O(\max(Np(m+n), n^3))$
SOFIA-IS	Simplex method	$O((m+p)m^2)\ p<n$	$O(p^3)$ where $p<n$
Graph-IS	Simplex	$O((m+n)m^2)$	$O(n^3)$

Computational Analysis

To evaluate the computational efficiency of Graph-IS with other algorithms, apriori analysis [4] is needed for Graph-IS. Table 7 presents the time complexity of isotonic separation and its variants and it reveals that Graph-IS guarantees to solve the LPP in polynomial time and it is mandatory to apply isotonic separation on large data set.

Findings

Theoretical, experimental and time complexity analysis show that Graph-IS is not only significant in classification performance but also it is able to solve the linear programming problem. The proposed graph-IS outperforms its counterparts EIS and MeHeIS-CPSO in classification performance. The conjecture for the superior performance is the ability to provide near optimum solution for the LPP and feature selection technique which is adapted for extracting isotonic features. Histogram based feature selection technique selects isotonic features as well as extends the isotonic regions in a feature space and reduces misclassifications. Even though the proposed histogram-based feature selection algorithm increases the size of the LPP, graph-IS labels the nodes or data points in polynomial time and faster than other variants of isotonic separation.

CONCLUSION

Graph-IS provides a graph-based framework for the isotonic separation method for classification. It can be applied to problems where isotonic consistency exists between features and class label. The proposed Graph-IS transforms the LPP into a DAG and obtains boundary points by mining the graph to extract bipartite graphs. These boundary points are used for classifying the unknown test data.

Experimental and statistical results show that Graph-IS significantly resolves the drawback of feature extraction in isotonic data and proposes another dimension of isotonic separation using graphs.

Plethora of topics that remain to be explored in the future include evaluating the Graph-IS in various domains such as internet content filtering, mail spam filtering and other publicly available large datasets. Spectral analysis can also be done on DAGs for solving LPP in isotonic separation. Graph-IS can also be generalized for multi way classification. In addition, the problem of finding the unknown isotonic consistency conditions for features constitutes a future research problem. Parallel or distributed architectures for solving LPP of isotonic separation will also be studied in future.

REFERENCES

[1] Ahuja, R. K., Magnanti, T. L. & Orlin, J. B. (1993). *Network Flows.* Prentice-Hall, Englewood Cliffs, NJ.

[2] Chandrasekaran, R., Ryu, Y. U., Jacob, V., et al. (2005). "Isotonic separation." *INFORMS Journal on Computing*, *17*(4), 462-474.

[3] Christopher JCB. (1998). "A Tutorial on Support Vector Machines for Pattern Recognition." *Journal of Data Mining and Knowledge Discovery*, *2*, 121-167.

[4] Cormen, T. H., Leiserson, C. E., Rivest, R. L. & Stein, C. (2001). *Introduction to algorithms.* MIT Press and McGraw Hill, New York.

[5] Dantzig, G. B. & Thapa, M. N. (1997). *Linear programming 1: Introduction*. Springer-Verlag, pp. 549–552.

[6] Deb, K. (2001). *Multiobjective Optimization Using Evolutionary Algorithm.* John Wiley & Sons Inc., New York.

[7] Fawcett, T. (2006). "An Introduction To ROC Analysis." *Pattern Recognition Letters*, *27*(8), 861-874.

[8] Goldberg, A. V. (1998). "Recent developments in maximum flow algorithms." In *Proceedings of Scandinavian Workshop on Algorithm Theory*, Springer-Verlag London, UK.

[9] Goldberg, D. E. (1989). *Genetic Algorithms For Search, Optimization and Machine Learning*, Addision Wesley.

[10] Hall, M., Frank, E., Holmes, G., Pfahringer, B., et al. (2009). "The WEKA Data Mining Software: An Update", *SIGKDD Explorations*, *11*(1).

[11] Han, J. (2005). *Datamining Concepts and Techniques*. Morgan Kaufmann Publishers Inc. San Francisco, CA, USA.

[12] Jacob, V., Krishnan, R. & Ryu, Y. U. (2007). "Internet content filtering using isotonic separation on content category ratings." *ACM Transactions on Internet Technology*, *7*(1), 1-19.

[13] Joachims, T. (1998). "Text Categorization with Support Vector Machines: Learning with Many Relevant Features." In: *European Conference on Machine Learning (ECML).*

[14] Joachims, T. (2002). *SVM Light Support Vector Machine*. http://svmlight.joachims.org/.

[15] Malar, B. & Nadarajan, R. (2013). "Evolutionary Isotonic separation for classification: theory and experiments." *Knowledge and Information Systems* Springer-verlag doi 10.1007/s10115-012-0579-5.

[16] Malar, B., Nadarajan, R. & Sai Sundara Krishnan, G. (2012). "Isotonic separation with an instance selection algorithm using softest: theory and experiments." *WSEAS Transactions on Information Science and Applications*, *9*(11), 350-367.

[17] Malar, B., Nadarajan, R. & Gowri Thangam, J. (2019). "A hybrid isotonic separation algorithm for training Evolutionary Isotonic separation for classification: theory and experiments." *Knowledge and Information Systems* Springer-verlag doi 10.1007/s10115-012-0579-5.

[18] Merz, C. J. & Murphy, P. M. (1998). "*UCI Repository of Machine Learning Databases*" Department of Information and Computer Sciences, University of California, Irvine.

[19] Monteiro, R. & Adler, I. (1989). "Interior Path following primal-dual algorithms. part II: Convex quadratic programming." *Mathematical Programming*, *44*, 43–66.

[20] Quinlan, J. R. (1993). *C4.5: Programs for Machine Learning.* Morghan Kaufman, San Mateo, CA.

[21] Ryu, Y. U. & Yue, W. T. (2005). "Firm bankruptcy prediction: Experimental comparison of isotonic separation and other classification approaches.", *IEEE Transactions on Systems, Man, and Cybernetics, Part A*, *35*(5), 727-737.

[22] Ryu, Y. U., Chandrasekaran, R. & Jacob, V. S. (2007). "Breast cancer detection using the isotonic separation technique." *European Journal of Operational Research*, *181*, 842-854.

[23] Watters, C. B. & Shepherd, M. (2003). "Support Vector Machines for Text Categorization." In: *Hawaii International Conference on System Sciences*, IEEE Computer Science Society.

[24] West, D. B. (2003). *Introduction to Graph Theory.* Prentice Hall of India.

In: Computing Paradigms for Smart Healthcare ISBN: 978-1-53618-619-2
Editors: B. Vinoth Kumar et al.

Chapter 6

CONVOLUTION NEURAL NETWORK: AN OVERVIEW IN MEDICAL IMAGE ANALYSIS

B. Padmapriya*, PhD, L. Abinaya, K. Pavithra, D. Roshini and L. Sugantha Sundari

Department of Biomedical Engineering,
PSG College of Technology, Coimbatore,
Tamil Nadu, India

ABSTRACT

The Deep Learning refers to multilayered Artificial Neural Networks. It has been considered one of the most effective tools over the past few decades, and has become very popular in literature because it has the efficiency to handle huge quantities of data. The Convolutional Neural Network (CNN) is one of the most common deep neural networks. It takes its term from the operation of linear mathematics that exists among matrixes named convolution. CNN has the "neurons" arranged

* Corresponding Author's Email: bpp.bme@psgtech.ac.in.

much like those of the frontal lobe, the region responsible for visual stimuli perception in humans and other animals. The neuron layers are structured in such a way that they cover the entire visual field avoiding the traditional neural network problems. CNN uses a device much like a multilayer perceptron built to meet reduced criteria for processing. A CNN layer is composed of an input layer, an output layer and a hidden layer that includes convolutional layer, fully connected layer, pooling layer and non- linear layer. In machine learning problems the CNN has excellent results. Especially in applications related to classification of the image and processing, the outcomes are remarkably impressive.

Keywords: CNN, artificial neural network, linear mathematics, convolution, neurons, multilayer perceptron, machine learning, deep neural network

INTRODUCTION

Evolution of CNN

In this chapter, you will learn about Convolutional Neural Network (CNN) is a state-of-art technology, branch of Deep Learning and its applications in medical Image processing. Neural networks become popular in recent years. It is currently developing a field that grabs the attention of youngsters and research scholars. Many researches and developments are going on to optimize this field. The first neural network designed is perceptron. Multilayer perceptron forms the bases for the Convolutional Neural Network. LeNet5 is the first CNN architecture build by YannLeCun in the year 1994 for the classification of handwritten numbers. Processing higher resolution images with CNN is computationally complex and requires high computational resources like GPUs and TPUs. Before the advent of GPUs and TPUs, CNN is at its infantry.

ImageNet is a challenge platform that is a repository of an image dataset with 15 million labeled high-resolution images and approximately 22,000 classes. From 2010, ImageNet Large Scale Visual Recognition

Challenge (ILSVRC) has been conducted annually. ILSVRC is a part of the ImageNet dataset with 1.3 million training images, 50,000 validation images and 100,000 testing images; about 1000 categories. The ultimate aim of this competition is to improve Computer vision techniques. For the first time ImageNet classification challenge was won by AlexNet Architecture with the classification accuracy of 84.7% in 2012 [1]. It beats all traditional handcrafted image classification algorithms. AlexNet is the first Convolutional Neural Network to use GPUs for accelerating deep learning training time. AlexNet, designed by Alex Krizhevsky, is considered as one of the most influential papers published in computer vision.

ZFNet proposed by Zeiler and Fergus, won the ImageNet ILSVRC 2013 with a validation error rate of 16.5%. It is the slightly modified version of AlexNet with the difference in filter size of 7X7 which is 11X11 in AlexNet [2]. This increases the accuracy of the model. It uses softmax as the classification layer (softmax layer will be explained later in the chapter).

GoogLeNet also called Inception, is the winner of ImageNet ILSVRC 2014 with a top-5 error of 6.67% and was proposed by Google. This network was designed based on LeNet with the difference that it used batch normalization, RMSprop as cost function and image distortion [3]. It takes advantage of several small convolutions to reduce the number of parameters to 4 million.

Following Inception, VGG16 and VGG19 network architectures, designed by K. Simonyan and A. Zisserman with less parameter compared to AlexNet hence reducing training time. VGG16 has about 138 million parameters [4]. This model achieved 92.7% accuracy in ImageNet competition 2014, becoming the runner up of ImageNet ILSVRC 2014. The training went for weeks, using NVIDIA Titan Black GPUs.

Subsequently, in 2015, ResNet Architecture was proposed by Kaiming He, Xiangyu Zhang, Shaoqing Ren and Jian Sun. Multi-version of ResNet was proposed with the name ResNet XX, where XX denotes the number of layers in the architecture. ResNet18 architecture has 11 million trainable parameters. ResNet152 achieves a high accuracy of 95.51%. The accuracy achieved by ResNet200, ResNet101 ResNet50 architectures is 95.51%, 93.95% and 93.29% respectively. Despite of increased number of layers, ResNet architectures are less complex compared to previously proposed architecture. It follows a new methodology of Residual learning which means skipping some subsequent layers and hence fine-tuning the output from previous layers.

Consequently, Dual Residual Swap Out Network (DRSN) and SENet won ImageNet ILSVRC 2016 and 2017. Hence, gradually Convolutional Neural Network (CNN) emerged to vision the computer Systems and its milestones are shown in Figure 1.

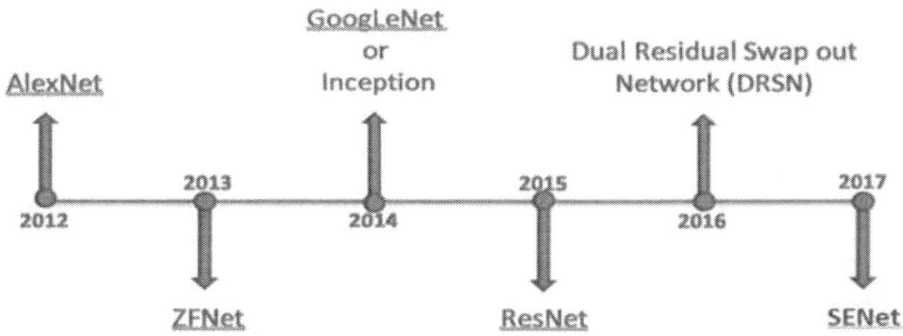

Figure 1. Milestones of CNN in ImageNet ILSVRC Challenges.

Google introduced Google Colab in 2014. It is a web-platform, uses Python as a coding language to develop machine learning-based applications with GPU and TPU support. It allows training the machine learning models with GPU support and hence decreasing the training time. It has inbuilt machine learning and deep learning APIs. It has a time limit of 12-hour usage per day.

Artificial Neural Networks

Before understanding about Convolutional Neural Network, let us know about the Artificial Neural Network. It is the replica of the Human Brain System in which millions of neurons are internally connected.

Information is passed from one neuron to the other through synapses. Likewise, in the Artificial Neural network, we have neurons connected in the form of layers. Perceptron is the first designed neural network. The simple architecture of a single layer perceptron is seen in Figure 1.2(a) [5].

Here X1, X2,..., Xn are the inputs. It can be in the form of records in spreadsheet (.xlsx or .csv file format) or Image data. W1, W2, ...,Wn are the weight values which is a numerical value adjusted by Backward propagation (Backward propagation is discussed later in this chapter) to reduce the error value. C1 and C2 are the two classes. Y value is calculated from the formula mentioned in the above figure. Activation function helps in determining the class of the input data. The output of the perceptron is the single class value for the input data given to the network. Following a single layer perceptron, the concept of a multilayer perceptron developed. The architecture of the multilayer perceptron is given in Figure 2 (a).

Multilayer perceptron is a feed forward artificial neural network consists of an input layer, an output layer and one or more hidden layers. Each layer made up of n number of neurons represented as a circle in the above Figure 2 (b) [5].

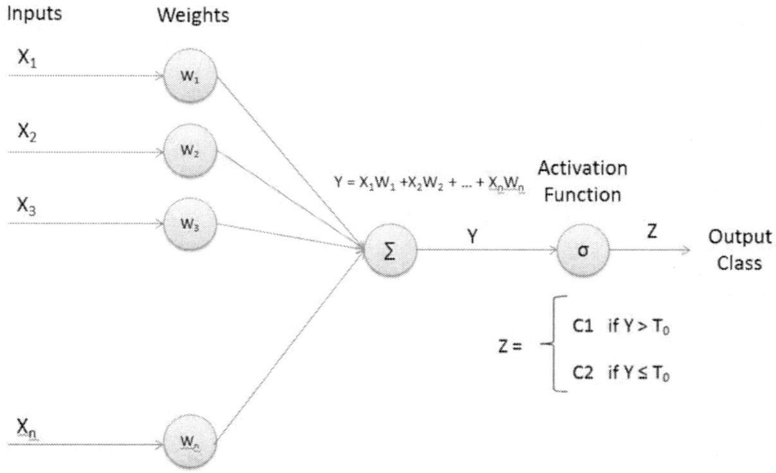

Figure 2 (a). Simple Architecture of Single Layer Perceptron.

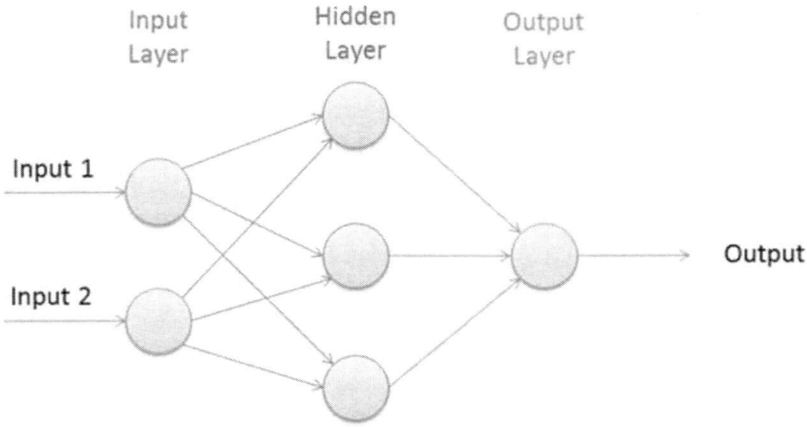

Figure 2 (b). Architecture of Multilayer Perceptron.

CNN

Convolutional Neural Network (CNN) is a subset of the Deep Learning technique. It plays an important role in Computer Vision. It is an efficient Computer Vision algorithm used in many medical image processing, pattern recognition and interpretation. It is a mimic of the Human Visual Cortex. The main advantage of CNN is that it required less pre-processing while traditional methods include hand engineering. Convolutional nueral networks use convolution instead of simple matrix multiplication (detailed working is discussed later in the chapter). CNN makes use of mathematics operation convolution to extract features from the dataset during training and in the testing phase, neurons get activated when the extracted features are found in the test image. CNN architecture is also called a neural network model.

There are two different types of learning: Supervised and Unsupervised. In *Supervised learning*, both the input image and output class are fed into the CNN model for training. It is used for image classification and image segmentation. Classification of Dog and Cat is an example of image classification in supervised learning. The dataset used in CNN consists of an input image labeled as Cat or Dog. If there are two classes in the classification it is called Binary Class Classification. Classification with more than two classes is called multiclass or categorical classification. In *Unsupervised learning*, only input image is fed into the model. Hence this learning is used in association or grouping of data. Grouping fruits as apple, orange or mango based on color feature is an example of unsupervised learning. The example of supervised and unsupervised learning can be referred in Figure 3(a) and (b) [7].

Now let us discuss the two primary terminologies in Artificial Neural Network, Forward Propagation and Backward Propagation.

The flow in which the inputs are fed through the successive network layers in the forward direction is called *forward propagation*. The input of one hidden layer is the output of the previous layer; flow is always from the first layer to the last layer.

After forward propagation, backward propagation occurs. Initially weight values are randomly initialized. In *backward propagation*, these weight values get adjusted to minimize the error. How these weight values are adjusted is decided by the Gradient Descent Algorithm used in Neural Network. In the coding perspective, Gradient descent algorithm is termed as an optimizer.

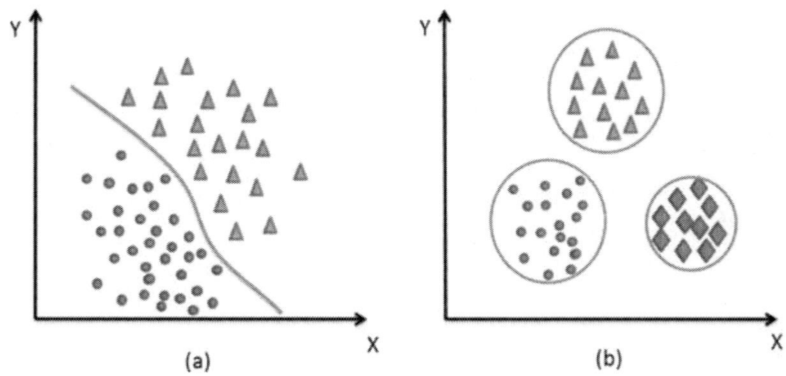

Figure 3. Example of (a) Supervised learning (b) Unsupervised learning.

CNN Terminologies

Any application with CNN undergoes three phases: Training phase, validation phase and testing phase. About 60%, 20% and 20% of the dataset is used for training, validation and testing phase respectively.

Training Phase

Forward and Backward propagation occur in the training phase. The model learns the features of the input dataset. The forward and backward propagation of all training dataset is called as one epoch. The number of epochs can be defined. The number of images fed through the network is defined as batch size. Increasing the batch size decreases the number of steps in the epoch. The correctly classified image to the total number of images gives the training accuracy. Weight values are updated only in the training phase. Mean Standard Error (MSE) indicates the deviation of true value and the predicted value and can be calculated as in equation (1).

$$MSE = \frac{1}{n}\sum_{i=1}^{n}\left(\left(Y_i - \hat{Y}_i\right)\right)^2 \qquad (1)$$

where n denotes the number of datasets, Y_i denotes the true value, $\hat{Y}_i$ denotes the model predicted value.

Parameters like epoch, batch size, learning rate, number of layers defined in a network are called hyper parameters. It helps in increasing the model accuracy (learning rate is discussed in Gradient Descent).

Validation Phase

At the end of every epoch, after the training phase, validation occurs. The Validation dataset is validated with the weight values updated in every epoch. It helps in determining if our model is learning in each epoch. If validation accuracy is very less than the training accuracy, then the model is said to overfit. When both validation accuracy and training accuracy is very less, then the model is underfit. Model with high accuracy in training and validation is said to be the best fit. The model doesn't learn if the validation accuracy remains constant for every epoch. A learning CNN model will have increasing validation accuracy.

Testing Phase

After training and validation, the modified weight values are saved in .h5 or. pb format. The input image is fed into the saved model to predict the class of the input image.

The testing accuracy and testing error are calculated correctly based on the predicted output class. Confusion Matrix is plotted for testing to understand the exact correct prediction of the dataset.

Confusion Matrix

The Confusion matrix is the tabular form that visualizes the classifier performance. From the confusion matrix, the specificity and sensitivity of the model can be calculated. The 2x2 confusion matrix is seen in Figure 4 [8].

The Sensitivity of the classifier determines how often the model correctly predicts the true value. It is calculated using the formula:

$$Sensitivity = \frac{TP}{TP + FN}$$

The Specificity of the classifier determines the ability of the model to correctly predict a false value. It is calculated using the formula:

$$Sensitivity = \frac{TN}{TN + FP}$$

An efficient model will have high sensitivity and high specificity.

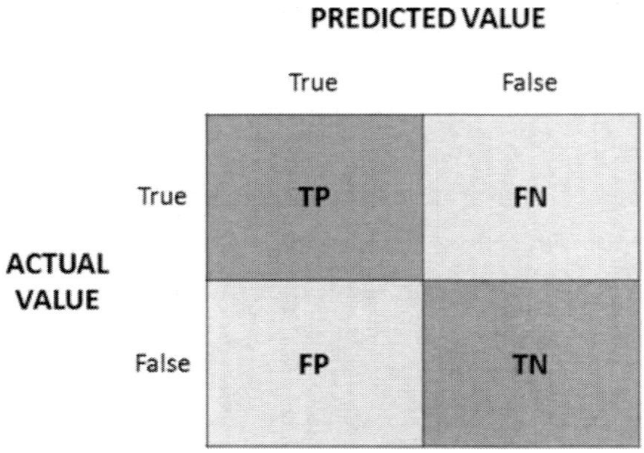

Figure 4. Confusion Matrix 2 x 2 Classification.

True Positive (TP) – Actual label is True, the model predicted as True
False Negative (FN) – Actual label is True, the model predicted as False
False Positive (FP) – Actual label is False, the model predicated as True
True Negative (TN) – Actual label is False, the model predicted as False

Transfer Learning

Transfer learning is a newly developed technique to improve the model accuracy. It is a means of transferring the knowledge gained by one model to another model with the help of weight values [8]. In other words, instead of initializing weight values randomly, this approach initialize weight value of a pre-trained network trained for other classification which is related to our application. This also helps in reducing the training period.

Activation Function

The activation function is a nonlinear function that is applied before the output from one layer is fed to the subsequent layer. Each layer can have an individual activation function. There are several activation functions and in the future the count may increase.

Sigmoid or Logistic Activation Function

Sigmoid activation curve is an S-shaped non-linear function. The output value of the layer is substituted in the equation specified in the Figure 5. The resulting value is fed to the subsequent layer. The output of the sigmoidal function ranges from 0 to1.

Softmax functionis a logistic activation function, used as an output layer for multiclass classification. Vanishing gradient is the drawback of sigmoidal activation function.

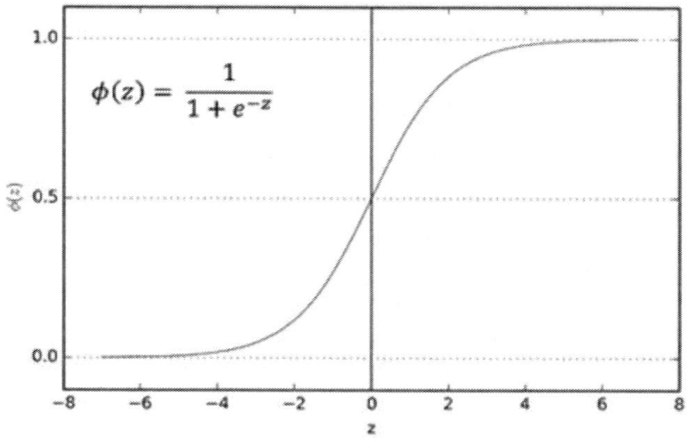

Figure 5. Sigmoidal activation function graph.

Tanh Activation Function

Tanh function is a nonlinear function with an S - shaped curve. The resulting layer output is passed through this function and fed to the next layer. The output values range from -1 to +1. This function is mainly used for binary class classification. It overcomes the problem of vanishing gradient in a sigmoid function. It overcomes the problem of vanishing gradient faced by sigmoid function. The equation and the graphical representation are seen in Figure 6.

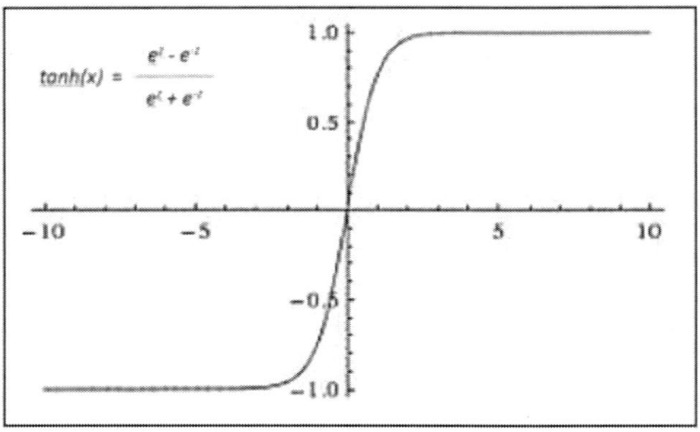

Figure 6. Tanh activation function graph.

ReLU Activation Function

Rectified Linear Unit (ReLU) is the commonly used activation function. Negative values are made zero in this function and positive values are fed as such to the next layer and is seen in Figure 7. Some weight values are not modified during backward propagation. It may lead to dead neurons. This limitation has overcome in LeakyReLU.

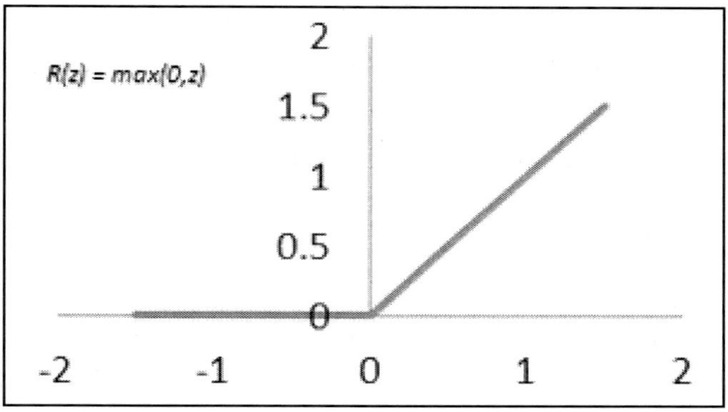

Figure 7. ReLU activation function graph.

Leaky ReLU

To overcome the limitations of ReLU, Leaky ReLU is introduced. The range of ReLU is increased in Leaky ReLU from -∞to +∞. Instead of making negative values to 0, the magnitude of the value is reduced, which is used to overcome dying neuron and vanishing gradient.

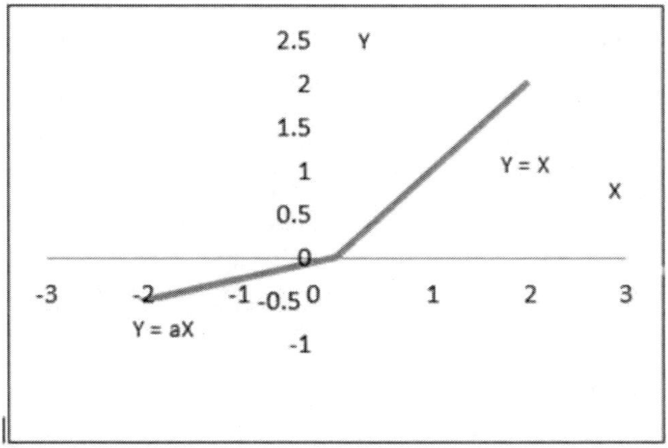

Figure 8. Leaky ReLU activation function graph.

From the above Figure 8, it is inferred that negative values are not made 0 as such. These are some of the activation functions commonly used in the CNN model.

CNN Layers

Complex and efficient architecture is built by stacking various layers and it is important for classification. The most common layers of CNN are explained further.

Convolutional Layer

Convolutional layer is the first neural network layer well known for the analysis of visual imagery and it is the foremost layer architecture given for input data. It extracts distinct features in the input feature map. Automatic learning of many filters in particular training or testing datasets under many constraints and modeling problems is the main advantage of a convolutional neural network. Highly unique and specific feature can be revealed anywhere on the input images is the outcome of a convolutional layer [10].

A convolution is the simple use of a filter to input data which results in an activation. Feature map is nothing but the map of activation, which is evaluated with the repeated use of the same filter to input data. Using the input data which is acquired from small squares, it learns the significant features of the image and maintains the relationship between the pixels. It is one of the essential layers to give the best accuracy. The advancement of computer vision on deep learning is mainly due to the convolution algorithm. When compared to the other layers its preprocessing time is low. Here the filter and input image or data is convolved to gain the feature, thereby forming an activation map Figure 9.

The important aim of the convolution operation is to detect high-level features of the input data. ConvNets need not be meant for only one convolutional layer. Initial layers are significant in adapting the low- level features followed by additional layers, capturing high-level features that collect wholesome details and features of images in the dataset. Convolutional layer is responsible for two sorts of results to the operation depending upon whether the dimensionality increases or remains the same. Comparing to the input, the convolved feature is reducing its dimensionality is called valid padding, whereas the operation is vice versa in case of the same padding [11].

Input

1	2	3	5	2	3
7	6	2	4	8	9
1	3	4	1	3	7
3	2	1	3	2	5
2	6	7	9	8	4
4	3	1	7	3	2

Filter

1	0	-1
1	0	-1
1	0	-1

Output when stride = 1

0	1	-4	-9
4	7	-6	-13
-6	-2	-1	-3
0	-8	-4	8

Output when stride = 2

0	-4
0	-4

Figure 9. Functionality of CNN layer.

Pooling Layer

The pooling layer which is also referred to as subsampling layer used to minimize the resolution of the features. Because of its destructive nature, pooling can be done in two ways as maxpooling and average pooling. In both types, the input is partitioned into non-overlapping two-dimensional spaces.

Alike a convolutional Layer, the Pooling layer is significant for diminishing the spatial size of the convolved Feature which reduces the computational power required to handle the data through dimensionality reduction. Dominant features such as positional and rotational invariant can be captured by this layer. Moreover, this layer is responsible for effective training of the model. The convolutional and pooling Layer, both form the ith layer of a Convolutional Neural Network which support in detecting minute low-level features in the image.

Max Pooling Layer

This layer operation depends on the calculation of maximum value in each patch of the feature map. Its main purpose is to down scale the input data by diminishing its measurement called dimensionality. The size of the pooling operations is always low when compared to the size of the feature map as shown in Figure 10.

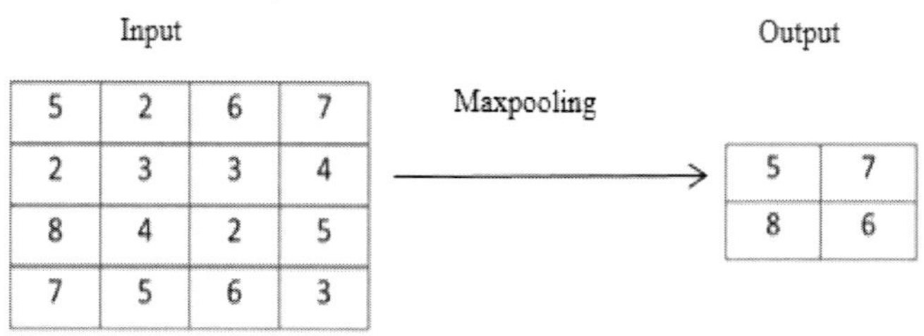

Figure 10. Functionality of Max Pooling layer.

It diminishes the parameter and computations in the network to overcome overfitting. The pooling layer divides the activation map into an equal set of rectangles and the largest value of each set is joined to form a Max Pooling layer. The most common size used for maxpooling operation is 2*2. Max pooling plays a crucial role in noise suppressant. Along with dimensionality reduction, it discards the noisy activities. While comparing the average pooling, max pooling performs better in case of de-noising.

Average Pooling

Average pooling performs calculation of average values on the selected patch of the activation map as shown in Figure 11. It applies non-linear down sampling on feature maps. The number of filters isn't affected. Average pooling finds its advantages in improving the efficiency [12].

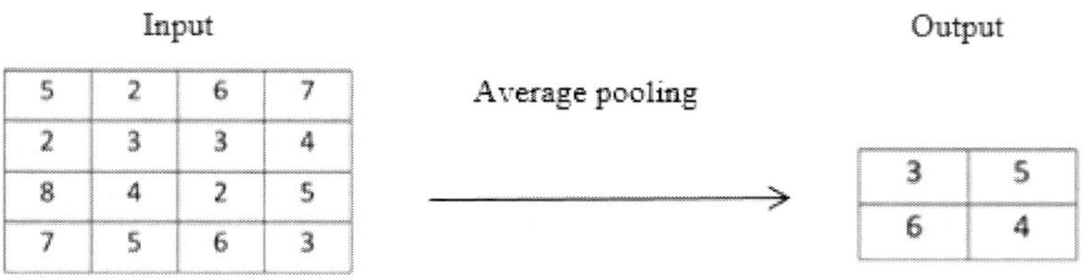

Figure 11. Functionality of Average Pooling layer.

Dropout layer

The objective of the dropout layer is to avoid overfitting by reducing correlation. It is one of the dynamic ways to perform a model operation in neural networks. Dropout layer finds its function in regularization techniques. It eliminates the extra parameters at each layer. It can dropout both hidden and visible units in the layer. But it has the drawback of passing information to the next layer merely.

It is one of the significant regularization techniques to reduce overfitting. Dropout layer is computationally cheap and improves generalization error in networks. The dropout layer can be implemented as a visible layer, hidden layer and also input layer, but it cannot be used as an output layer [13].

Flatten Layers

Flatten layers scale down the multilevel images into one-dimensionality without losing its valid features. It preserves the weight ordering when shifts from one input representative to another. It converts the whole pooled feature matrix into a separate column which is then provide into a network model. Flatten layers is used to combine convolutional and dense layer into a single layer which is then given to a neural network.

Dense Layers/Fully Connected Layer

Dense layer is the one which connects the input weight to the output weight. The dense layer uses linear operation. A fully connected layer often used as a final layer in the model. The outcome gets from the final pooling layer or convolutional layer is flattened, which is the converted into a one-dimensional array of vectors and it is combined to one or more dense layer. By learnable weight, a fully connected layer is responsible for connecting every input to each output. Mapping between the subset of layers to the final outputs can be done only after the completion of the feature extraction of the convolutional layer and down sampling of the pooling layer. After the mapping, the classification task will exist. The fully connected layer is followed by an activation function. It is important for learning the non- linear combinations of high-level features.

Batch Normalization

Batch normalization is a method helps in stabilizing the learning process and to adjust the pace and performance of the network model. It can reduce the number of training epochs to train the model. It diminishes the generalization errors [13].

Embedding Layers

Embedding layer is used to reduce or compress the input features in the dataset. It can be able to minimize the loss function and its output cannot be the mathematical function of the input. Mostly embedding layer is used for text data in neural networks.

APPLICATIONS OF CNN IN MEDICAL IMAGING

Radiology

CNN also finds its application in radiology such as image segmentation, image reconstruction, image classification, lesion detection. It is used in the classification of radiology free-text reports. It is also used to detect the type of fracture using radiographic images. It is used to detect the brain tumor from radiographic images.[17]

Image Tagging

Image tagging is a process of adding tags, labels or hints to the recognized things or faces with a certain feature that makes easier to identify an image. Google and amazon use this technique. It is used in the biometric system. CNN also finds its application in image segmentation and feature extraction.

Drug Discovery

Deep learning is also used in cancer drug repurposing. It is also used to develop a drug repurposing tool kit including repurposing for COVID19. It is used to identify the molecular pattern which is used in drug discovery. It is used in DTI (Drug Target Interaction) which is used in silicon drug discovery.

Dental

CNN is used in the precise classification of dental disease using RVG (Radio Visiography). CNN is also used in dental plaque quantification. CNN provides comparatively high results in dental plaque quantification compared to the manual method. CNN is also used in the cephalometric landmark detection in dental x-ray images.

Brain Tumor

Segmenting and detecting neoplasms are used in radiotherapy treatment. Manual segmentation of neoplasms is a time consuming task. CNN helps in segmenting neoplasms. CNN is not only used for detection, but also it is used for brain tumor classification. It is done based on the DWT fusion of MRI sequences [22].

METHODOLOGY

Data Augmentation

Existing methods for image augmentation can be classified very much into one of two specific categories: traditional, white-box or black-box methods based on deep neural networks. Throughout this section, we present briefly the classes of methods that have had the largest effect in the area of image synthesis and augmentation [18].

Traditional Transformations

This is the most common current data augmentation method being doing a combination of affine image transformation and color alteration. Defines the affine transformations: rotating, reflection, scaling (zoom in / out) and shearing in Figure. 12 (a).

In general, geometric distortions or deformations are used to increase the number of samples used to train deep neural models, to suit the size of the dataset, and to improve their efficiency, which is commonly used as affine transformations to increase the results for data increase but is still the subject of study. The most common methods are: equalization of the histograms, enhancement of contrast or brightness, white balance, sharpening and blurring and is seen in Figure 12(b) [18].

These methods are simple to understand, they proved to be fast, reproducible and reliable.

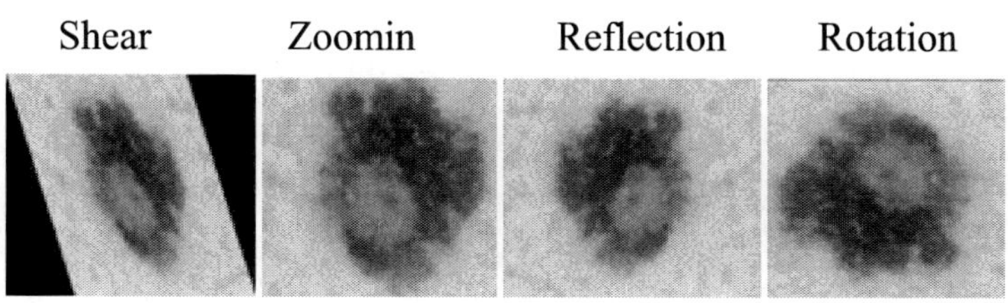

Figure 12 (a). Same image after different types of affine transformations.

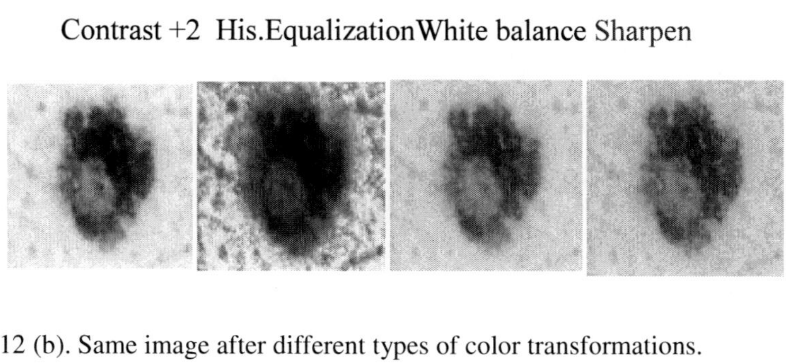

Figure 12 (b). Same image after different types of color transformations.

Generative Adversarial Networks

Generative Adversarial Network (GAN) is a relatively new and powerful tool which uses a min-max strategy to perform unsupervised generation of new images. GANs were considered to be incredibly useful in many different problems of image creation and editing, such as text- to – image synthesis, super resolutio (generating high-resolution image from low-resolution one), image-to-picturetranslation (e.g., converting drawings into images), mixing images (mixing selected parts of two images to create a new one), image painting (restoring lost image pieces).

The general concept of GANs is to use two adversarial networks (G(z) and D(x)), where one creates a photo-realistic image to deceive the other net (generator G(z)) equipped to help distinguish false images from true ones (discriminator D(z)). In other words, the role of the generator is to minimize cost (value) function V (D, G) (for instance, the maximum probability), while the discriminator maximizes it (Figure 13) [18].

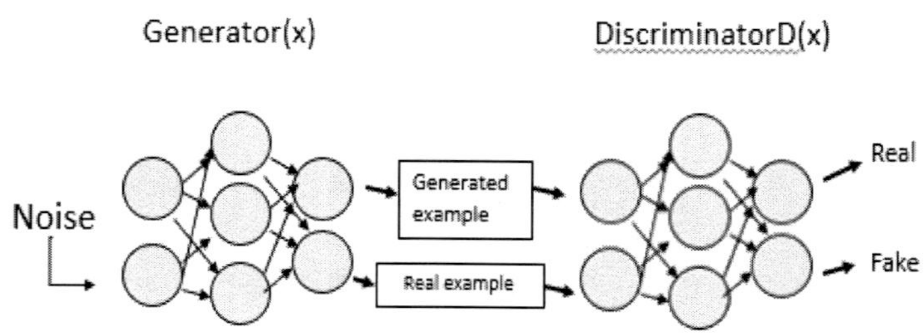

Figure 13. Simplified concepts of Generative Adversarial Network.

Texture Transfer

The aim of the texture transfer is to synthesize a texture from a texture-source image while constraining a content-source image's semantum content. This task aims to add a certain texture to a new image so that the original image's visual attributes, such as contour, shading, curves, strokes and regions, remain visible. Many traditional methods of texture transfer rely on the principle of resampling the texture into a given image of the content. The common technique called picture quilting for example is a way of synthesizing a new image by stitching together tiny patches of existing pictures.

The image augmentation methods currently being developed are not restricted to the conventional and CNN based methods. One of the interesting approaches is a random erasing technique that is quick and fairly easy to implement and yet gives good results in CNNs' ability to generalize. In the process one randomly paints a rectangle filled with noise in an picture that results in a change in the original pixels values [19]. Therefore the expansion of the dataset with images with various levels of occlusion decreases the chance of overfitting and makes the pattern sturdier.

Style Transfer

The style transfer method, that's closely related to texture and color transition, has recently begun to get more attention from researchers and even its already fading value in conventional methods is gradually growing. The style transfer aims in synthesizing a new picture that imitates the style of the data-source while the content-source image semantic material is restricted.

Feature Map

The feature map represents the output of one filter applied to the previous layer. A provided filter is drawn all over the previous layer, one pixel moved at a time. Each position causes the neuron to activate and the output is collected in the feature map. It is seen that if the receptive field is moved from activation to activation by one pixel, then the field will overlap with the previous activation by input values (field width - 1).

CNN's feature map shows the result of filters being applied to an input image. The feature map at each layer is the output of that layer. The purpose of seeing a feature map for a particular input picture is to try and obtain some understanding of what the CNN detects. Perhaps it can sense some of our target object's pieces, and not others, or the activations may die out on a certain layer. It is also important to note a common concept in Deep Learning directly, that early network layers track low-level features (colors, boundaries, etc.) and that later network layers track high-level features (figures and objects).

Let's see an example in which a convnet filter functions on the data, performs the convolution process and as a result we get a feature map. To get an output volume, we use several filters and we stack together the resulting feature maps.

Feature Map Visualization

The feature maps can be visualized to see how inputs are transformed, going through layers of convolution. The feature maps are often called as intermediate activations since the layer's output is called the activation. A volume of 3D is the output of a convolutional layer. The feature map's height and width of correspond to the dimensions, and each channel of depth is a different feature map encoding separate features. So we will plot each channel in a 2D image format to represent individual feature maps. It is pretty easy to visualize the feature maps. We pass through the CNN an input image and record the activation intermediate. Then we choose and plot certain feature maps at random.

The names for convolutional layers of VGG are: blockX_convY. For example, block3_conv2 is called second filter in the third convolution block. In this chapter, feature map of Retinal Image is studied. Lets have a look into the features that can be extracted using the model.

Figure 14 shows the damages caused to eye blood vessels due to Diabetic Retinopathy, eye abnormality which consequently leads to vision loss. Aneurysm, hemorrhage (blood leakage) and hard exudate are the features present in the image. Here is how one of the feature maps from the very first layer data (block1 conv1) appears.

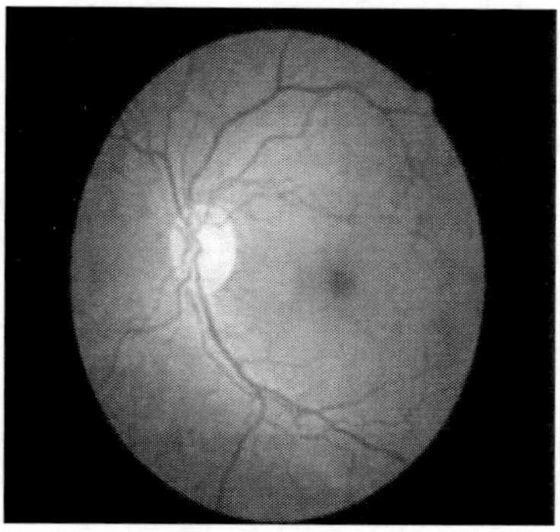

Figure 14. Retinal Damage due to Diabetic Retinopathy disease.

From the Figure 15 bright areas are the "activated" regions, which indicate the identified pattern, the model is searching for. This filter encodes a blood vessel pattern in the image. Multiple feature maps from a convolutional layer would be more useful to display, instead of looking at a single feature map. Let's see the feature maps which correspond to the first convolution of each block, the red arrows in the figure below.

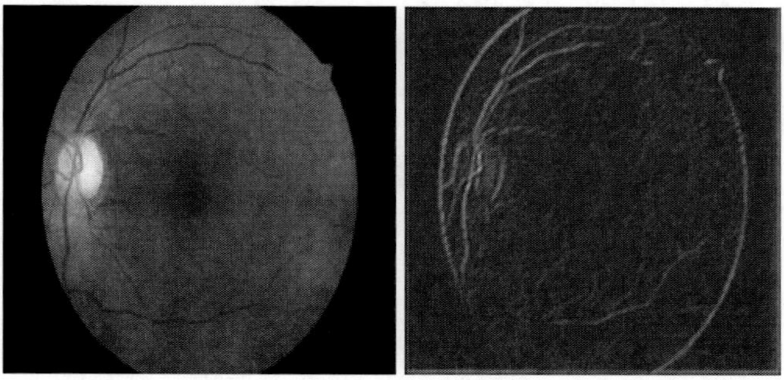

(a) (b)

Figure 15. (a) Funduscopic Retinal Image (Input image) (b) Result of first Conv Layer.

The Figure 15 (c) is the layers of the architecture. Now let us analyze how the images would transform on passing through these layers.

The following Figure 16 (a) shows 8 feature maps for each layer. Block1_conv1 contains 64 feature maps, since that layer contains 64 filters. In this figure, however, we visualize only the first 8 per row.

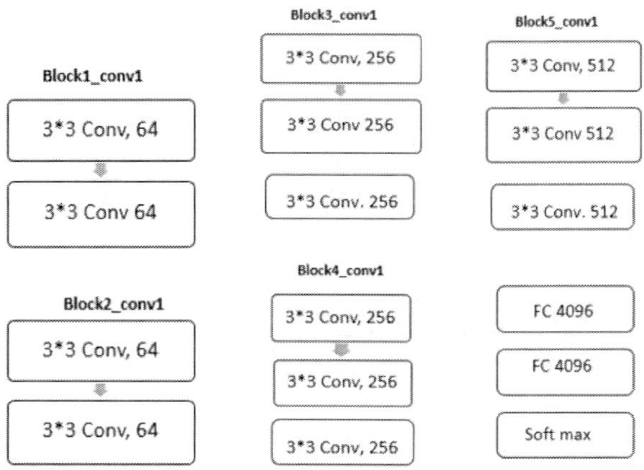

Figure 15 (c). Network Architecture.

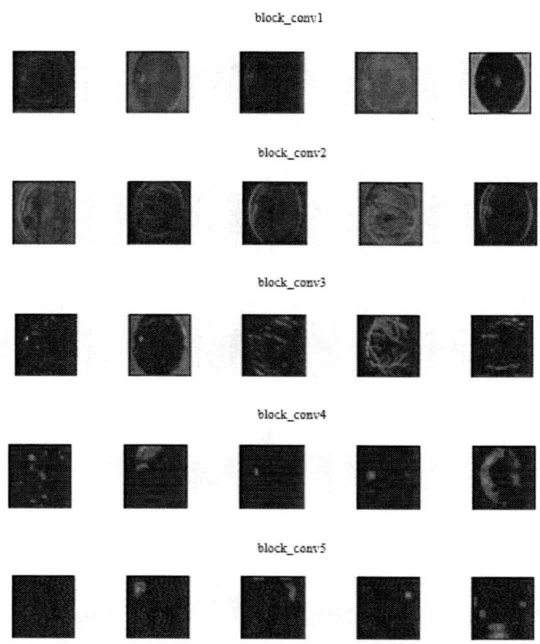

Figure 16 (a). First 5 feature maps of the retinal image.

block_conv1 block_conv2 block_conv3 block_conv4 block_conv5

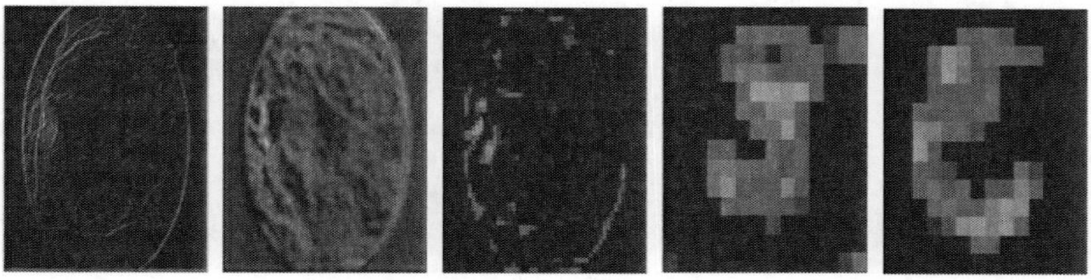

Figure 16 (b). First 5 feature maps of five convolutional layers

As we pass through the layers, there are few important views on the feature maps. To make it clearer, let's look at one map per layer of features.

Note: Feature Map count increases exponentially as the convolutional layer increases. Only first five Feature Maps are plotted above. There are as many as feature maps as filters. For e.g., If a network has 512 filters, then there are 512 feature maps for each convolutional layer.

The feature maps of the first layer (block1_conv1) (Figure 16 (b)) Leave most of the graphic info here. For CNN architectures the first layers typically serve as edge detectors.

The feature maps look less similar to the original picture and more of an abstract representation of that, as we move further into the network. It's because of that deeper feature map represents high-end concepts such as "blood vessels" or "blood leakage" whereas the feature maps of the basic edges and shapes. So, the deeper feature maps contain less picture information and more details about the image class. They still represent important features, but we are less able to view them visually.

As we go further, the feature maps become sparser, meaning that features are less detected by the filters. It makes sense because the first-layer filters detect basic shapes, and those are contained in each image. But as we get deeper, we begin to look for more complicated things such as "exudates" and they don't appear on every picture. This is why we see more maps as blank as we go deeper, with 8 filters per layer in the first example, (block4_conv1 and block5_conv1).

Gradient Descent Algorithm

Gradient descent is the prominent algorithm method to execute the operation of optimization and it is also useful for optimizing neural networks. Different algorithms are available for optimizing gradient descent. It is one of the methods to minimize the objective function in numerous machine learning algorithms. It is essentially helping in upgrading the parameters of the network model and it is computationally expensive.

Gradient Descent Variants

There are three main variants are available in this decent algorithm such as batch gradient descent, stochastic gradient descent and mini-batch gradient descent. Usage of data to compute its operation is varied in all three variants.

Batch Gradient Descent

Batch gradient descent is also called as vanilla gradient algorithm, responsible for computing the gradient of the objective function as regard of the parameter θ for the wholesome data input as given in equation 2.

$$\theta = \theta - \eta \cdot \nabla(\theta)\, J(\theta) \tag{2}$$

Batch gradient descent is preferred when the amount of dataset is limited in case of a huge dataset it cannot be preferred as it is computationally expensive. The main disadvantage of this descent is that doesn't apt for the memory space and slow. Calculating the gradients for the entire dataset in just one update is impossible as it does not allow the model to update to the next level. It can converge to global minimum and local minimum for convex and non- convex error surfaces [14].

Stochastic Gradient Descent

Stochastic gradient descent will take parameter upgrade for every individual training dataset example x(i) and label y(i) as in equation 3.

$$\theta = \theta - \eta \cdot \nabla(\theta)\, J\, (\theta; x(i); y(i)) \tag{3}$$

Because of re-computation of gradients, batch gradient descent will result in redundant computations for huge datasets whereas the stochastic descent will overcome this flatness by achieving one more upgrade at a time. That is why the stochastic method is typically faster and it has the capability of learning online. Due to frequent updates, the objective function of the image may get fluctuate. Convergence is the same as that of batch gradient descent. The Stochastic method rarely results in overshooting [15].

Mini-Batch Gradient Descent

Mini-batch gradient descent has a stable convergence because of the minimization of the variance of the parameter updates. It performs in an efficient way by computing the gradient. The size of generally used mini-batch ranges varied from 50 to 256 but it is not constant which may differ according to the various applications. Along with mini-batch descent sometimes stochastic gradient is also used.

Momentum Gradient Descent

Stochastic gradient descent has a drawback in handling the areas where curves of the surface are mostly steep in 1D than the other which is usually occurs around local optima. Momentum gradient descent is the only option that helps to reduce this issue. Importantly momentum technique can be worn to get faster convergence and to minimize oscillation.

Adam Optimizer

It is an optimization technique, updated algorithm of stochastic gradient descent procedure. It is computationally efficient and requires a little memory when compared to the other gradient descent algorithm. The extension of stochastic gradient descent is the Adam optimization technique which has many utilizations in computer language processing. In order to update network based on training data, this extension from classical stochastic gradient decent to the Adam optimization algorithm has occurred.

Adam has the advantage of combining two factors of stochastic gradient such as the adaptive Gradient Algorithm (AdaGrad) and Root Mean Square Propagation (RMSProp). The former one manages a parameter learning rate, which helps in improving performance on problems with sparse gradients and the later one is responsible for maintaining non-stationary problems like noise. Because of the faster results Adam optimizer used in the deep learning algorithm [16].

CASE STUDIES AND DISCUSSION

Detection of Melanoma Using CNN

Objective

Melanoma is one of the deadliest forms of skin cancer, which need an expert dermatologist for its detection. Early disease identification plays a vital aspect due to the effects caused by the disease. In addition to this, skilled and experienced dermatologists only can accurately diagnose melanoma. An automated system is required for early detection to preserve the time and effort. Physicians use the ABCDE method to detect melanoma. It means asymmetric, irregular border, non-uniform color, larger diameter and evolving of the mole are the features considered in the detection of melanoma. However, the accurate melanoma recognition is extremedifficult because of contrast difference varied between lesions and skin, visual comparison between melanoma lesions and normal. A Deep convolutional neural network can detect melanoma based on features like shape, color and diameter with less time. Resnet50 architecture is used along with some additional layers to build our neural network model.

Dataset

The training dataset has its importance in training the Convolutional Neural Network model since its accuracy relays on the dataset. Melanoma dataset is available on ISIC drive, a collection of quality controlled dermatoscopic images of skin lesions which has taken under various imaging conditions.

ISIC is an international organization, has a repository of skin images used to train clinicians and provides standard to melanoma diagnosis. They posted challenges along with the dataset to detect the presence of melanoma. Dataset downloaded contains approximately 16000 images and the sample images of melanoma and non-melanoma are given in Figure 17 (a) and 17 (b). Among them, 8904 for training 3562 for validation and 3561 images are used for testing.

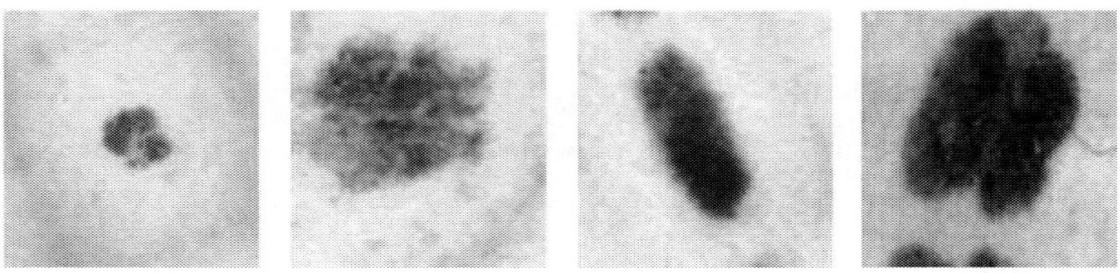

Figure 17. (a) Melanoma Images.

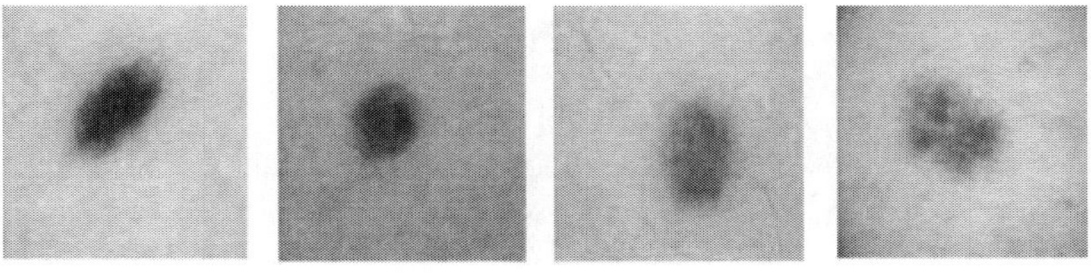

Figure 17. (b) Non- melanoma Images.

Pseudo Code

INPUT Collect Melanoma Dataset (ISIC)
Image preprocessing to remove noise in images
Construct Neural Network Architecture RESNET50s
START training **FOR** number of epoch
    INPUT image flow through CNN
predict image class as melanoma or non- melanoma
    Calculate loss value and accuracy for each epoch
    IF loss value and accuracy variation is positive
        COMMIT weight values
    ELSE
        RESET weight value updates
Calculate accuracy and loss metrics

Architecture

The architecture used is Resnet50 with some additional layers (flatten, dense, dropout) achieved high accuracy. The layers used and the parameters are shown in this Table 1.

Table 1. Architecture of Resnet50 with additional layers

LAYERS	PARAMETERS
2ResNet50	23587712
Flatten	0
Dropout	0
Dense	102761472
Dropout	0
Dense	2050

The following architectures are used for training such as Xception, Inception, MobileNet and VGG16. High accuracy is achieved in ResNet50.

Hyper Parameters

Weight values are initialized randomly and are updated by employing Adam Optimizer. The learning rate is specified at 0.0001. It is a binary class classification with two classes: Melanoma and Non-Melanoma.

Sigmoid Activation function is used to fire the neurons upon extracting the features. With the help of the GPU support in Google Colab, the model is trained with the ISIC dataset for 5 epochs. It takes 90 minutes of training and validation.

Results and Observation

The training and validation accuracy of the model is 97.57% and 93.53% respectively. The training and Validation loss of the network model is found to be 1.1727 and 1.9237 respectively.The loss metrics for each epoch is plotted as in the Figure 18.

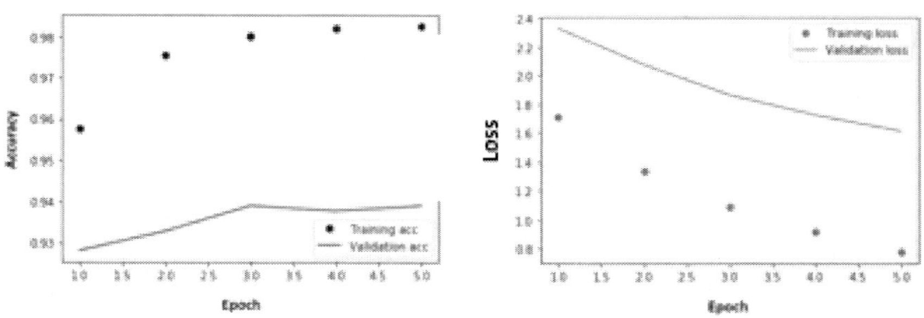

Figure 18. Accuracy and Loss graph for Validation and Training.

The Confusion matrix is the tabulation to estimate the performance of classification model. It consists of prediction labels in the X-axis and True Label or known values in the Y-axis to assess the accuracy, specificity and sensitivity of the trained model. The 2x2 confusion matrix for this case is shown in Figure 19.

Sensitivity defines the ability of the model to predict positive results for those with the disease. Specificity defines the ability of the model gives negative results for those without the disease. The sensitivity, specificity and accuracy can be calculated using the following equations 4, 5 and 6 respectively,

$$Sensitivity = \frac{TP}{TP+FN}\ X\ 100.. \tag{4}$$

$$Specificity = \frac{TN}{TN+FP}\ X\ 100 \tag{5}$$

$$Accuracy = \frac{TP+TN}{TP+FP+TN+FN}. \tag{6}$$

In this, the sensitivity and specificity of the trained model are calculated to be 84.73% and 100% respectively. The testing accuracy of the model is 92.36%.

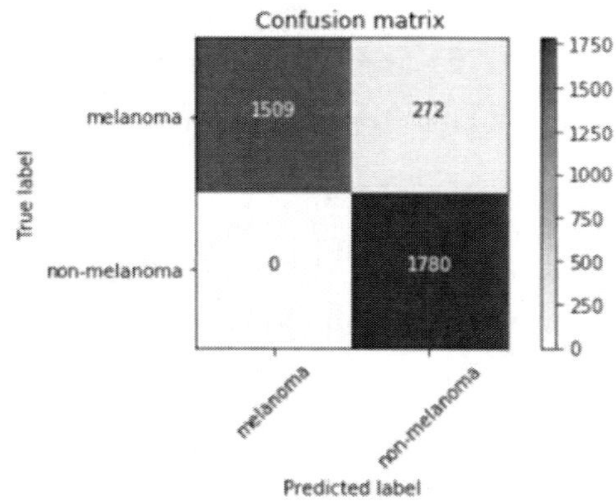

Figure 19. Confusion Matrix of the testing Model.

Diabetic Retinopathy Detection

Objective

Diabetic retinopathy is the long term complication of diabetes, which may lead to vision impairment if left untreated. The early stage of diabetic retinopathy has no symptoms. Only half of the people who are affected by diabetes are aware of diabetic retinopathy. This blindness can be prevented if it is diagnosed early. This can be done with the help of a screening test. The accuracy in disease detection depends on imaging modalities which is a time consuming task due to the manual effort of the experts. It can also be done with the help of some deep learningtechniques.

A Deep convolutional neural network is proposed to detect the severity level of the diabetic retinopathy, which relies on the presence of microaneurysm, exudates, neovascularization and hemorrhage. Clinicians categorized DR into 5 stages: Normal, Mild DR, Moderate DR, non-proliferative DR (NPDR) and proliferative DR (PDR). DCNN is a more complex architecture that helps to classify the stages of DR.

Dataset

The fundoscopic retinal image used for the project is taken from Kaggle which provides a huge number of high-resolution retinal images with various disease conditions. Both left and right eye fundoscopic images were provided. Ophthalmologist labeled each retinal image based on the severity as 0,1,2,3,4 for No DR, Mild, Moderate, Severe and ProliferativeDR respectively.

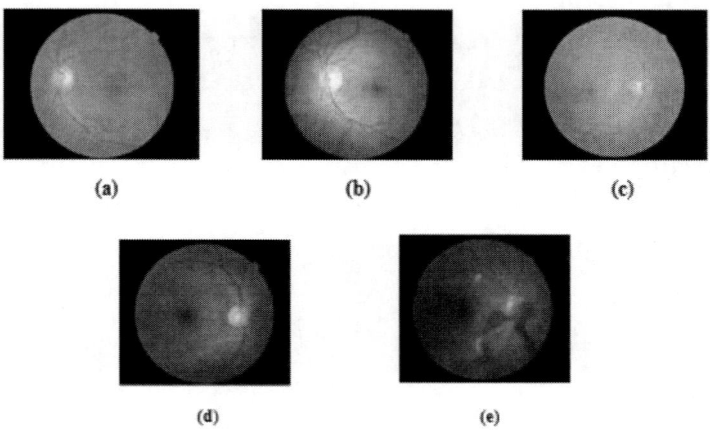

Figure 20. (a) No DR (b) Mild DR (c) Moderate DR (d) Severe DR (e) Proliferative DR.

This dataset provides around 80000 images, but we used 8242 images for training our model to reduce the training time and prevent overeating. Equal number images are taken with no DR and disease conditions like mild, moderate, non-proliferative DR and proliferative DR and a sample image of each type is shown in Figure 20. Along with the dataset an Excel spreadsheet is also available. The spreadsheet contains image names and respective labels.

Pseudo Code

INPUT Collect DR Dataset
Image preprocessing to remove noise in images
Data Augmentation
Construct CNN Architecture
START training **FOR** number of epoch
    INPUT image flow through CNN
predict image class as No DR, mild DR, moderate DR, severe NPDR or PDR
    Calculate loss value and accuracy for each epoch
    IF loss value and accuracy variation is positive
        COMMIT weight values
    ELSE
        RESET weight value updates
Calculate accuracy and loss metrics

Architecture

The network architecture used to train the model to classify the diabetic Retinopathy is given in Table 2.

Table 2. Architecture

LAYER	FILTERS	OUTPUT	PARAMETERS
Convolutional	32	128 X 128	896
Convolutional	32	126 X 126	9248
Max Pooling	32	63 X 63	0
DropOut	32	63 X 63	0
Convolutional	64	63 X 63	18496
Convolutional	64	61 X 61	36928
Max Pooling	64	30 X 30	0

Table 2. (Continued)

LAYER	FILTERS	OUTPUT	PARAMETERS
DropOut	64	30 X 30	0
Convolutional	64	30 X 30	36928
Convolutional	64	28 X 28	36928
Max Pooling	64	14 X 14	0
DropOut	64	14 X 14	0
Fully Connected	12544		0
Dense	512		6423040
DropOut	512		0
Dense	5		2565

Data Augmentation

Before the dataset is given to the convolutional layers, preprocessing has to be done to remove the unnecessary noises. The fundoscopic images were taken from different types of cameras which results in the varied and noisy retinal images. Hence, data augmentation such as image resizing, rotation, random shift, flipping has been done.

Classification

The classification has been done with the epoch of 15, an initial learning rate of 0.0001, batch size of 32 into five different classes as mild, moderate, non-proliferative DR, proliferative DR and normal. Computationally efficient Adam optimizer is used.

Results and Observations

The overall accuracy of the model is 73.49% and overall loss is 0.8875. The graphical representation of training loss, training accuracy, validation loss and validation accuracy are given below in the Figure 21.

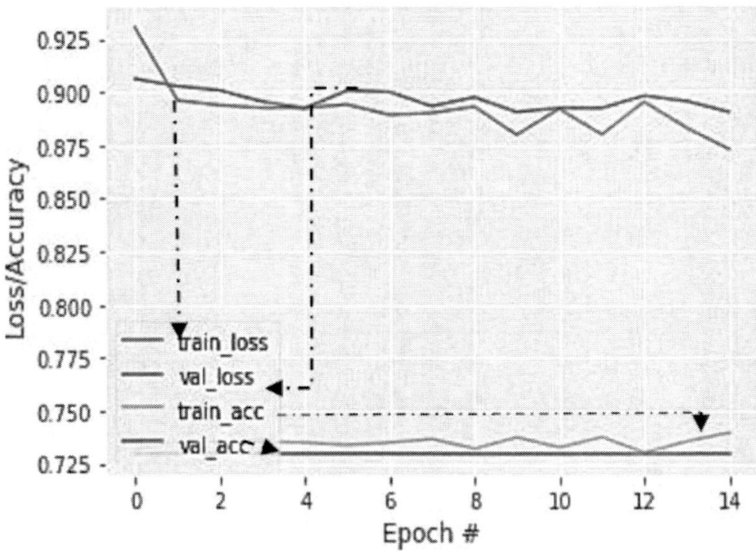

Figure 21. Training loss and accuracy of diabetic retinopathy detection.

The trainable parameters used in the network are 6,565,029. Moreover, the model is a lightweight with a minimal number of convolutional layers used.

WBC Classification

Objective

The white blood cell count is an important indicator of health and is important for many diagnostic tests. Currently, doctors utilize expensive automated counters. Therefore, it would be helpful to have an automated way to detect and count WBCs. Detecting WBCs is the first step for achieving this goal. Blood-borne disease diagnosis also requires identification and characterization of blood samples from patients. Automated ways of identifying and classifying blood cell subtypes have significant applications in medicine.

This can be achieved using Deep Learning. The Convolutional Neural Network is known in Deep Learning as the suitable network to get the features. Hence CNN architecture is used to obtain the features of the different blood cells and the trained model can classify the images based on the obtained distinct features. These features include size, color, shape and the presence of granules.

Dataset

The dataset to train the model is collected from Kaggle. BCCD dataset contains 12,500 blood cell images. There are four folders in which 3000 images are grouped based on cell types.

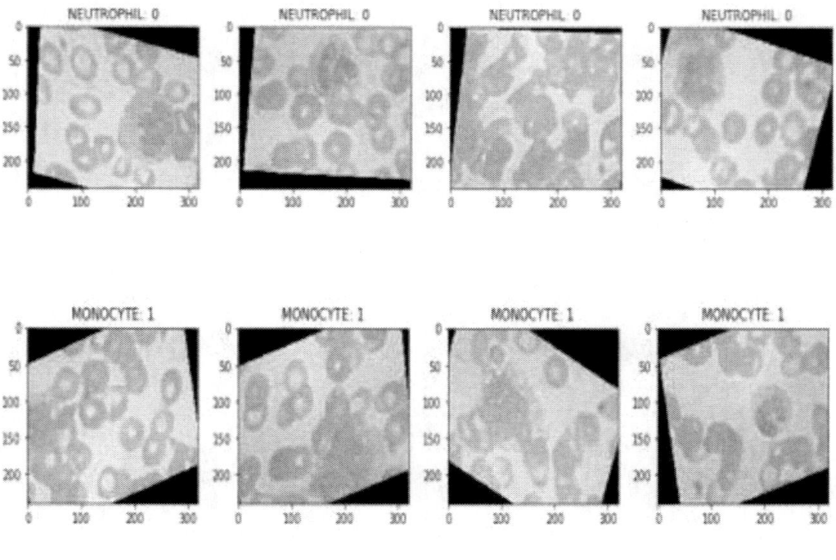

Figure 22. Four different types of WBCs.

The types of cells are Eosinophil, Lymphocyte, Monocyte, and Neutrophil and their sample dataset is shown in the Figure 22.

Pseudo Code

INPUT Collect WBC image Dataset
Image preprocessing to remove noise in images
Data Augmentation
Construct VGG16 Neural Network Architecture
START training **FOR** number of epoch
    INPUT image flow through CNN
predict image class
    Calculate loss value and accuracy for each epoch
    IF loss value and accuracy variation is positive
        COMMIT weight values
    ELSE
        RESET weight value updates
Calculate accuracy and loss metrics.

Architecture

The network model used is VGG16 with some additional layers and is shown in the Figure 23. VGG16 architecture achieves the best results, outperforming a single GoogLeNet by 0.9%. This network is defined by its simplicity, because it uses only 3×3 convolutional layers. Maxpooling is performed to reduce volume size. A Softmax classifier is accompanied by two fully-connected layers.

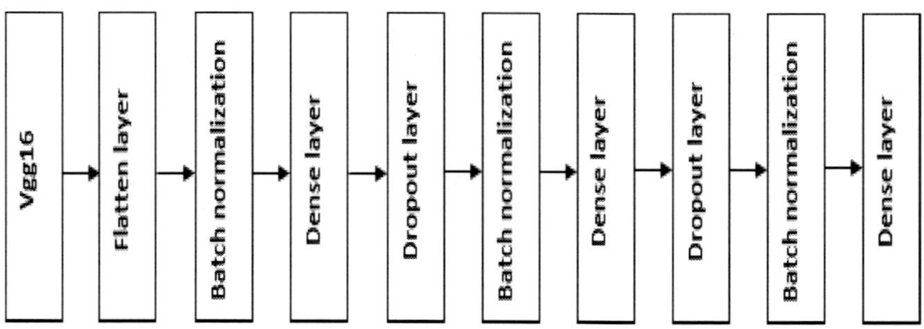

Figure 23. Model Architecture.

Hence, in addition to the VGG16 network model some additional layers such as dense, dropout, flatten layers are used.

Data Augmentation

The dataset should be pre-processed before proceeding into any neural network model. Hence, data augmentation is done. The images are rescaled, rotated, randomly zoomed, horizontal and vertical flipping is done.

Classification

CNN model is trained using 12500 images with 15 epochs. The batch size to train the data is 20 and the learning rate is initialized to 1e-4. Classification is done under the classes of four different classes. The Adam optimizer is used here.

Results and Observations

The training and validating accuracy are 81.47% and 86.85% respectively, and the accuracy is also plotted as shown in the Figure 24.

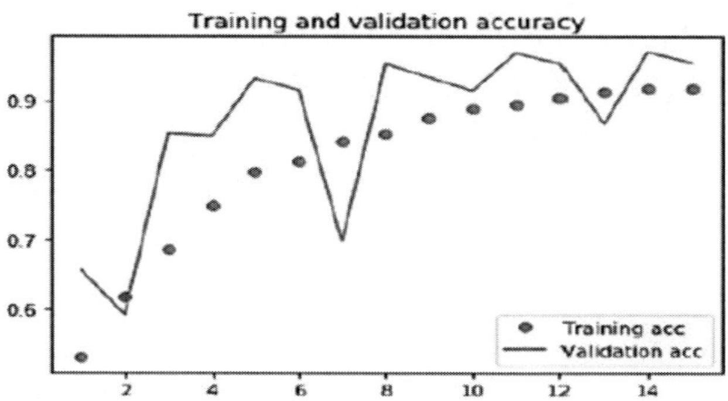

Figure 24. The training and validating accuracy.

Hence this model has increased accuracy, it also serves as an indicator that reflects even the small infection within the body and helps the hematologist to identify the abnormal increase in WBC called leukocytosis.

Retinal Disease Classification

Objective

Classification of the retinal diseases is an important problem in Computer-Aided Diagnosis (CAD) for clinical applications. OCT (Optical Coherence Tomography) has become an incredible imaging technique for non-invasive evaluation of various retinal diseases, such as aiding the diagnosis of CNV (Choroidal Neo Vascularization), DME (Diabetic Macular Edema), and DRUSEN. However, with the measure of image data created with the advanced OCT technology expanding, the feasibility of traditional OCT evaluation in clinical practice has gotten irrational. Thus, computerized discovery of retinal issues on retinal OCT pictures would be of huge advantage that could push ophthalmologists to all the high proficiently assess and treat eye-related diseases. With the help of CNN, automatic classification of retinal diseases can be performed.

Dataset

The OCT images are downloaded from Kaggle which contains high-resolution images used to train the model. Kaggle is an online association towards machine learning practitioners and data scientists which provides a huge number of high-resolution datasets. The OCT (Optical Coherence Tomography) images are taken from Kaggle for training and testing. Around 84,500 are downloaded from Kaggle. The downloaded images are in four folders as DME, CNV, DRUSEN and NORMAL.

Almost 90% of a dataset that is 83,484 OCT images is used as a training dataset and the remaining 1167 images which are collected from Kaggle are used to test and validate the model. The above Figure 25 is the sample dataset of four classes downloaded from Kaggle.

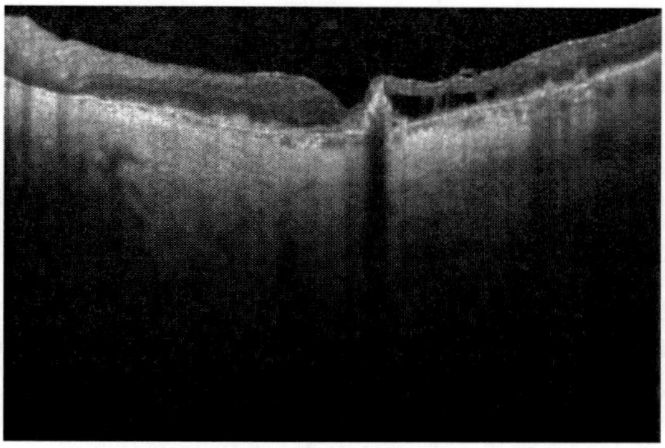

Figure 25. Sample dataset of retinal images

Pseudo Code

INPUT Collect OCT image Dataset

Image preprocessing to remove noise in images

Data Augmentation

Construct VGG16 Neural Network Architecture

START training **FOR** number of epoch

INPUT image flow through CNN

predict image class as CNV, DME, Drussen or normal

Calculate loss value and accuracy for each epoch

IF loss value and accuracy variation is positive

COMMIT weight values

ELSE

RESET weight value updates

Calculate accuracy and loss metrics

Architecture

VGG stands for Visual Geometry Group. VGG16 is one of the pre-trained models that give high accuracy to date and it contains 16 to 19 layers. This architecture shows better accuracy compared to others in this application.

Data Augmentation

Data Augmentation is a way of increasing the dataset with the help of the existing dataset. It includes cropping, padding, shifting, zooming and flipping of images. These multiplied images are used for training. Keras library provides Image Data Generator classes to perform data augmentation. It overcomes overfitting and increases accuracy. It makes the model robust to accurately classify rotated or shifted OCT images.

The images are resized, rotated, randomly zoomed, brightness levels are changed, and horizontal and vertical flipping is done.

Comparison with Other Models

Accuracy can likewise be increased by selecting the best pre-trained model. Various pre-trained models such as Xception, Inception V3, Resnet, Inception resnet, and VGG16 are compared. VGG16 has the highest training, Validation and testing accuracy, therefore VGG16 along with additional layers are used to train the dataset.

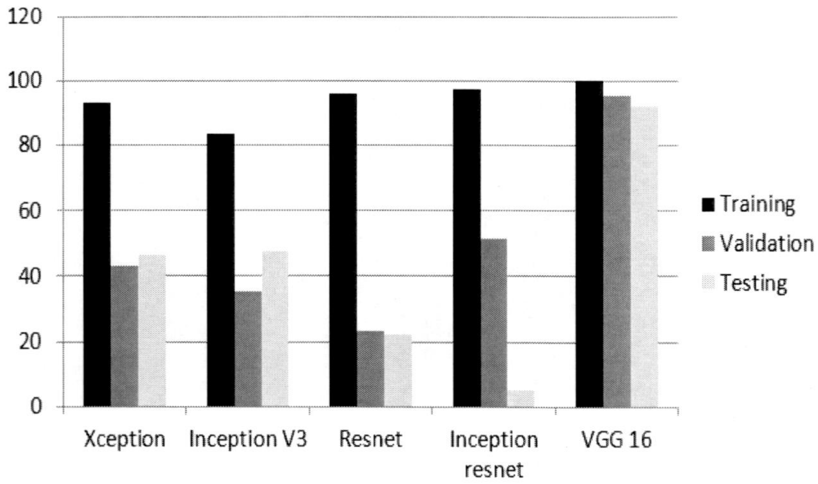

Figure 26. Comparison with other architectures.

The above Figure 26 represents the accuracy of various pre-trained models with additional layers such as Convolutional, Maxpooling, Dropout and Flatten.

Results and Observations

The model is trained with the Kaggle dataset for 50 epochs with the training time of15 minutes for training and validation. The training and validation accuracy of the model is 100% and 95.36% respectively as shown in Figure 27.

The sensitivity and specificity of the trained model are calculated to be 84.73% and 100% respectively. The accuracy is further increased by image augmentation which is a part of preprocessing, is performed and feature visualization for each class is also performed.

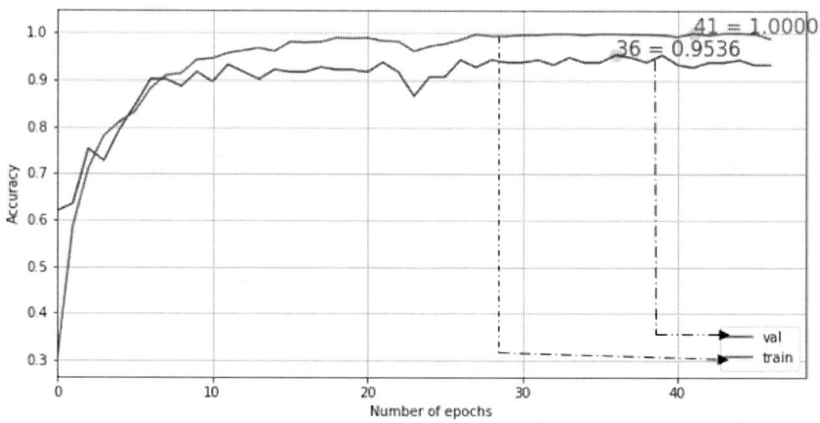

Figure 27. Training and validation accuracy of VGG 16 Architecture.

The neural network model is built using predefined VGG16 architecture along with some additional layers. Since the developed model has a high accuracy it tends to be utilized for classifying various conditions of retinal damage.

Conclusion

CNN has been influential and it has been increasingly growing in the field of medical imaging. We have addressed about the history of CNN and various levels of CNN in depth. Artificial Neural Network is explained using single layer perceptron design followed by multilayer perceptron design. The difference between the types of learning such as Supervised and Unsupervised are discussed. The two main terminologies on artificial neural network are forward and backward propagation is clarified. The difference between three main phases that any CNN model undergoes are training, validating, testing is discussed.

The visualization of classifier performance can be analyzed using confusion matrix and sensitivity and specificity formula is also highlighted. Transfer learning which the newly developed technique is explained briefly. Activation function is used to decide whether that neuron should get fired for that input, same as the rim the Activation functions used are clearly stated. An effective architecture is built by stacking multiple layers and discussing the unique feature of each layer.

Feature visualization task may be used to see how the input data is converted and flowing across the convolutional layers. Optimization can be done using one of the prominent algorithms called Gradient descent algorithm. An example coding is also given using the MNIST dataset. The top five applications of CNN in medical imaging are also discussed. From the four case studies, hope the implementation of CNN in medical imaging is understood.

References

[1] Krizhevsky, Sutskever I., and Hinton G. 2012. *"ImageNet Classification with Deep Convolutional Neural Networks,"* Papers.nips.cc.

[2] Matthew D. Z., and Fergus R. 2014. "Visualizing and understanding convolutional neural networks." *Proceedings of the 13th European Conference Computer Vision and Pattern Recognition*, Zurich, Switzerland.

[3] Szegedy, Vanhoucke V., Ioffe S. Shlens J. and Wojna Z. 2016. *"Rethinking the Inception Architecture for Computer Vision,"* arXiv.org.

[4] Simonyan, Karen, and Andrew Zisserman. 2014. "*Very deep convolutional networks for large- scale image recognition*." arXiv preprint arXiv: 1409.1556.

[5] Chollet F. 2016. "*Xception: Deep Learning with Depth wise Separable Convolutions,*" Open access.thecvf.com.

[6] Sun C., Shrivastava A., Singh S., and Gupta A. 2017. "*Revisiting Unreasonable Effectiveness of Data in Deep Learning Era,*" Arxiv.org.

[7] Yalniz, Jégou H., Chen K., Paluri M., and Mahajan D. 2019 "*Billion-scale semi-supervised learning for image classification,*" arXiv.org.

[8] Li X., Pang T, Xiong B, Liu W, Liang P., and Wang T. 2017. "Convolutional neural networks-based transfer learning for diabetic retinopathy fundus image classification," 10th International Congress on Image and Signal Processing, *BioMedical Engineering and Informatics* (CISP-BMEI), Shanghai.

[9] Kingma D., and Ba V. 2014. "*Adam: A Method for Stochastic Optimization*" International Conference on Learning Representations. Sciencedirect.com.

[10] Saha S. 2018. "*A Comprehensive Guide to Convolutional Neural Networks—the ELI5 way*", towardsdatascience.com.

[11] Brownlee. 2019. "*A Gentle Introduction to Pooling Layers for Convolutional Neural Networks,*" Machine Learning Maste.

[12] Srivastava N, Hinton G, Krizhevsky A, and Sutskever I. 2014. "*Dropout: A Simple Way to Prevent Neural Networks from Overfitting,*" Research gate.

[13] Dogo E, Afolabi O, Nwulu N., and Twala B. 2018. "*A Comparative Analysis of Gradient Descent-Based Optimization Algorithms on Convolutional Neural Networks,*" Research gate.

[14] Yu Y., and Liu F. 2019. "Effective Neural Network Training with a New Weighting Mechanism- Based Optimization Algorithm," In *IEEE Access,* vol. 7, pp. 72403-72410.

[15] Yamashita R., Nishio M., Do R. K. G. 2018. "Convolutional neural networks: an overview and application in radiology." *Insights Imaging* 9, 611–629.

[16] Mikołajczyk A., and Grochowski V. 2018. "*Data augmentation for improving deep learning in image classification problem,"* International Interdisciplinary PhD Workshop (IIPhDW), Swinoujście.

[17] Chen H., and Cao V. 2019. "Deep Learning Based Data Augmentation and Classification for Limited Medical Data Learning," *IEEE International Conference on Power, Intelligent Computing and Systems (ICPICS),* Shenyang, China.

[18] Wilamowski B. M. Dec. 2009. "Neural network architectures and learning algorithms," In *IEEE Industrial Electronics Magazine*, vol. 3, no. 4, pp. 56-63, doi: 10.1109/MIE.2009.934790.

[19] Deng J., Dong W., Socher R., Li L., Kai Li and Li Fei-Fei. 2009. "ImageNet: A large-scale hierarchical image database," *IEEE Conference on Computer Vision and Pattern Recognition*, Miami.

[20] Yang J., and Li J. 2017. *"Application of deep convolution neural network,"* 14th International Computer Conference on Wavelet Active Media Technology and Information Processing (ICCWAMTIP), Chengdu.

In: Computing Paradigms for Smart Healthcare ISBN: 978-1-53618-619-2
Editors: B. Vinoth Kumar et al.

Chapter 7

ADVANCES IN COMPUTATIONAL METHODS FOR CANCER DIAGNOSIS AND RESEARCH

Subramanian Vidyalakshmi*[*], *PhD
Department of Biotechnology, PSG College of Technology,
Coimbatore, Tamil Nadu, India

ABSTRACT

Cancer is a highly devastating disorder, affecting people of all ages and regions. A major hindrance to cancer treatment is the very high heterogeneity and complexity of cancer even within the patient's cells. Hence, there is significant variability in patients' responses against generalized cancer therapy. This opened up the leads for precision and personalized medicine in cancer. Precision medicine aims at targeting patient-specific tumor cells. This is achieved by accurately capturing clinical variations in tumor patients, and categorizing the patients into clinically relevant groups for targeted treatment options. Initially, patients were stratified based on the clinical symptoms, information from histopathology reports, environmental factors and certain limited genetic factors. With the advent of high throughput sequencing technologies,

[*] Corresponding Author's Email: vids21@gmail.com.

massive data is available on gene expression levels, mutation types, epigenetic information and copy number variations. These multi-omics information needs to be combined with clinical parameters, pathology reports and staging information in patients. For the clinicians to decide on tailor-made treatment options, the data has to be carefully analyzed and converted to clinically relevant outcomes. These multidimensional data sets demand tools like Artificial Intelligence to train such variations and decode genotypic – phenotypic relations and hence could help towards disease prediction, outcome and treatment modalities. This chapter summarizes recent advances in AI tools applied in cancer diagnosis and research for disease prediction and biomarker discovery.

Keywords: artificial intelligence, cancer big data, NGS, multi-omics, Digital pathology, TCGA

INTRODUCTION

Personalized medicine is a rapidly advancing new branch of medicine, which works on approaching a disease while accounting for an individual's variability factors like genetics, lifestyle, environment, etc., This allows clinicians to offer tailor-made treatment options, to suit an individual or a group of similar patients. Cancer is a global problem, affecting millions of people every year. Although significant efforts and money are spent towards research in cancer medicine, it is still an area of active analysis due to the complex nature of the disease and its heterogeneity. Hence, working towards precision medicine for cancer therapy is a critical task, accounting for the multidimensional data that has to be taken into account. This calls for excessive computational power and powerful algorithms for patients' stratification and clinical decision making. Various deep learning algorithms have been put into practice to reduce dimensionality in cancer big data. Significant improvements have already been made in the area of digital pathology, wherein pathology slides are digitized and clinically relevant decisions are made by applying suitable deep learning algorithms. Another area of active research is the application of AI in cancer genomics. With the completion of the human genome project, massive improvements have been made in the sequencing strategies. These high throughput methods have resulted in the data explosion of genomic, transcriptomic, epigenomic information on cancer. This chapter walks through the complex data on cancer and AI tools researched towards manipulating cancer data for decision making by clinicians.

The chapter is organized under the following sections:

- Big data in cancer
- Computing advancements in cancer 'Omics'
- AI in digital imaging and
- Conclusion.

BIG DATA IN CANCER

Cancer is a leading health problem globally [1], and multiple factors lead to cancer. As a result of this, there is a high heterogeneity recorded in cancer [2]. This heterogeneity makes cancer a complex disorder and hence accounts for the poor prognosis of many cancers. It is well known that cancers of various tissues occur due to the dysregulation of a plethora of genes involved in multiple metabolic pathways. Hence it is expected that a genome, transcriptome, or epigenome analysis of cancer gives rise to a complex representation of the disease state. Even, cells from various sites within a cancer patient have shown variations in the omics pattern.

Genomic information became popular after the completion of the Human Genome Project, which took 13 years to complete (1999-2003). This was a major public-funded initiative, involving more than 200 collaborators from around the Globe [3]. The effort involved Sanger basedsequencing platform to analyze information on the 20,000 and more genes and many interesting observations were made thereafter. Later, it was found that this sequencing method was less efficient and expensive. After years of extensive research, Next Generation Sequencing platforms were introduced [4]. Several NGS technologies are available as on date like Illumina HiSeq, SOLiD, Ion Torrent, Nanopore, SMRT, etc., With these technology platforms, it is relatively easy for the scientific community to generate sequencing information at a relatively low cost.

A transcriptome represents all the messenger RNAs that are produced by a cell at any point in time. Popular methods to generate transcriptome information include microarray and RNA sequencing [5,6]. Microarray techniques measure the expression levels of genes in two samples by comparing the fluorescent intensity generated after hybridization to the appropriate probes immobilized onto the microarray slides. RNA seq generate sequencing information and hence reports unknown sequences also.

A methylome data gives information about the methylation status and hence the "ON" and "OFF" state of any gene at that point. Copy Number Variations (CNV) explain the variations in the number of copies of genes.Mutation data reports the type of mutations like Single Nucleotide Polymorphisms (SNPs), Insertions- Deletions, etc., in any region of the genome.

Apart from the omics data discussed above, there are various clinical observations like the metabolic status of an individual, other biochemical parameters, histopathology images in case of solid tumors, imaging information, non-clinical parameters like age, other demographic factors, other disease conditions, lifestyle factors and environmental factors that are recorded for any patient.

Are these data considered as big data? The answer to this question is "yes". There is plentiful data in cancer medicine. Apart from this information, cancer data also comprise of whole-genome data which exceeds 100 GB. Computational analysis of these is highly data-intensive. The processed data includes trimmed reads from sequencing information, image analyses and genotyping information. These usually occur as structured data.

Hence, there is a massive data available per patient. Yet, the patient cohort having similar data storage is very less.Therefore, there is an imbalance between the depth of information versus cohort size in cancer data. This is even more pronounced in rare cancers like head and neck cancers. Nevertheless, several Machine learning approaches are routinely being researched to overcome this bias. This demands the availability of cancer data in publicly available repositories. National Cancer Institute (NCI) has launched various portals for the quick availability of cancer research data.

The NCI Genomics Data Commons (GDC) is a data science facility that links cancer-specific data with various analytical tools. It is a single point of data available from various data portals like The Cancer Genome Atlas (TCGA), tumor alterations relevant for genomics-driven therapy (TARGET) and the Genomics Evidence Neoplasia Information Exchange (GENIE).GDC helps towards data downloading, sharing and storage through various tools, publicly available.

Apart from this, NCI also provides cloud infrastructure for efficient data analysis, intending to advance efficient cancer research.

TCGA is a public-funded repository, which generates and catalogs cancer omics signatures. More than 30 tumors have been analyzed and the sample numbers exceed 20,000. TCGA has over 2.5petabytes of genomic, transcriptomic, epigenomic, mutation and proteomics data [7].

With the massive data, it becomes inevitable for AI tools to find its place in cancer data mining and discovery.

COMPUTING ADVANCEMENTS IN 'CANCER OMICS'

AI and ML are revolutionizing the way cancers are identified and grouped. A major challenge in managing cancer is the early detection of tumors, as this drastically increases the number of available treatment options, increases patient survival and hence improving the quality of life in the survivors.

Commonly used tests to diagnose cancer include imaging tests, endoscopy procedures and tissue biopsies.

Imaging tests include CT scans, MRI, X – rays, ultrasound imaging and other such radiographic analysis. Various endoscopic procedures like colonoscopy, bronchoscopy, thoracoscopy and the like have been used for the detection of various cancers. Biopsy tests include fine needle biopsy, excisional biopsy, cystoscopic biopsy, etc.

Various AI tools have been applied in imaging analysis for early and precise diagnosis of cancer. A detailed review on imaging is summarized in the next section.

Early detection of cancer is hindered by the high degree of variability among patients in the presentation of symptoms and the molecular heterogeneity of cancers themselves. Traditionally used Statistical techniques are highly unreliable and inaccurate. Hence, the use of ML techniques is imperative in cancer diagnosis. ML is used to generate predictive models that apply logical rules from already available patient-specific information.

Apart from the advent of AI applications in imaging and digital pathology, AI offers solutions to manipulate complex multi-omics cancer data. This has helped clinicians to offer personalized treatment options to patients [8-10].

NGS techniques have helped to get an overview of the complete genomic profile of cancers. With the developments in similar high throughput sequencing techniques platforms, there is an exponential growth in the availability of massive Biological data. The data include multi-layered studies to integrate data from DNA sequencing, RNA sequencing, epigenome, proteome, microbiome, metabolome, etc., An integrated approach is essential to understand the complexity of cancer. When efficiently utilized, these data have the potential for the identification of highly sensitive biomarkers for cancer diagnosis, prognosis and survival outcomes.

NGS techniques are increasingly being adopted at the clinical setup. There are several FDA approved cancer panels like Oncomine, Dx Targettest, MSK – Impact and so on.

One of the largest databases – TCGA illustrated the utility of NGS in discovering novel tumor pathways and potential classification strategies (The Cancer Genome Atlas Research Network, 2012) [11]. Way et al., (2018) [12] have applied the ML approach to the TCGA dataset to detect

Pan-cancer Ras pathway activation. They have integrated data from various platforms like Illumina RNA Seq, mutation calls, CNV from the TCGA Pan-cancer Atlas project. The massive data thus generated was trained using a supervised elastic net penalized logistic regression classifier[13].

Rendleman et al. [14] have used Multivariate Imputation by Chained Equation (MICE) to predict survival outcomes by applying variances from clinical variables from the TCGA dataset. RNA expression profiling data was used and the method reduced the computational cost and time.

Tranchevent et al. [15] applied deep neural networks, which work on a graph-based method for feature extraction from high throughput omic datasets of neuroblastoma patients. In this study, the ML model was applied to reduce the features by applying graphical topology. This was followed by predictive models to predict the outcome of patients in the training dataset. DNN outperformed Support Vector Machine (SVM) in prediction. DNN could capture complex features and was able to predict with very high accuracy and sensitivity.

Ma and Zhang [16] have applied Multi-view factorization Auto Encoder (MAE) to integrate multi-omics data to relate molecular features and clinical features from TCGA datasets.

Apart from these, various clustering methods are available to analyze multi-omics data (Table 1). It is mandatory to integrate such a large number of data from small sample numbers. Hence, the concatenation strategy has been applied to omics data.The simplest method is early integration, which is derived from concatenating omics matrices and applies clustering algorithms over this matrix, e.g., i- Cluster [17]. This utilizes the joint latent variable model for integration. Early integration methods suffer various disadvantages: If the normalization is not done properly, it might result in biased weightage to omics data. Second, it does not relate the distribution of data in various omics platforms. Finally, data dimensions are increased, as it considers individual omics data and finally clusters them. Especially multi-omics data suffer from overfitting.

A way to alleviate this problem is by regularization or adding additional constraints to reduce dimensionality. LASSO (Least Absolute

Shrinkage and Selection Operator)creates a regularization model in which the number of features with non zero effects on the set is minimal. i-cluster uses the LASSO regularization feature. LRACluster regularization is based on probabilistic models. The feature distribution is decided by a latent sample representation. This model was used to analyze pan-cancer data from TCGA [18].

In late integration, each omics matrix is individually clustered and later integrated [19]. The advantage of late integration is that any existing algorithm can be used for clustering. Algorithms that are shown to work well with any single omic data can be used independently to analyze that data and later these can be clustered. So there is no need to create a unified new algorithm.

COCA was used in a pan-cancer TCGA analysis to find how different tumors cluster and whether the clusters could be matched with the originating tissues. Each omic data was clustered separately by this algorithm and then the concatenation was done. The algorithm initially clusters single omics data, such that the$m$'th omic has$c_m$clusters. For sample$i$in omic$m$clustering is given as a binary vector$v_{im}$of lengthc_m, where$v_{im}(j) = 1$ if$i$belongs to cluster$j$and 0 otherwise. On the other hand, Bruno et al., [20], have used a probabilistic latent fusion semantic algorithm for clustering. The above two methods work well for any single omic analysis.

PINS [21] integrates cluster by determining the connectivity matrices obtained from individual omics. The matrices are then averaged to a single connectivity matrix. The clusters are then split into smaller clusters. Perturbations are generated by adding Gaussian noise to the data. PINS require original data for modeling.

Meanwhile, similarity-based methods employ similarities or distances across samples and use this information for data clustering. Wang et al., [22] have used Similarity Network Fusion (SNF) on mRNA expression, methylome data, etc., from TCGA. This model utilizes networks of samples for integration, rather than considering individual observations. This thus creates a patient network and is the first of its kind to be used in Biological data analysis. SNF involves two major steps: Generation of the patient network, followed by clustering of networks by a nonlinear combination method. They have shown that SNF could derive meaningful annotations from small sample size and multiple genes. This could also be trained to evaluate tumor subtype stratification. Table 1 summarizes the various multi-omics clustering methods.

Table 1. Various multi omics custering methods and their features

Method	Tool	Advantages	Reference
Early integration	LRACluster – R Structured sparsity-Matlab	Unsupervised clustering, abe to handle multiomics data faster and efficiently	Wu et al., [18] Wang et al., [23]
Alternate optimization	MV k-means, MV EM	Successive iteration improves the objective function value	Bickel et al., [24]
Late integration	COCA Late fusion using latent models PINS	Can be used even when raw omic data is unavailable	Bruno et al., [25] Nguyen et al., [21]
Similarity-based methods	Spectral clustering generalizations– Matlab SNF	Noise correction by multiple iterations	De Sa, [25],Kumar et al., [26],Chikhi, [27]; Li et al., [28] Wang et al., [29]
Deep learning methods	Neural networks, A variant of CCA, early integration and middle integration approaches	Multiple paratmeters could be easily integrated	Andrew et al., [30] Chaudhury et al., [31]

Rappoport and Shamir [32] have done extensive research on various multiview methods and benchmarked them with the data from TCGA. The authors have demonstrated that rMKL- LPP outperforms other methods in clinical enrichment, and MCCA and multi NMF performed better over others in predicting survival. The authors have also developed neighborhood-based multi-omics clustering (NEMO), a novel algorithm for multi-omics clustering and it also performs better even when there is a missing omics data.

For identification of commonly occurring co differential genes, Multiview NMF had been attempted [33]. A graphregularized version of multiview NMF was employed to encode genomic data. Manifold regularization was given as manifold alignment. The method was applied to data from TCGA, with multi-omics datasets. GMvNMFwas shown to be a better performer than the other methods.

In another study [34], graph regularization was used in the generation ofa regularized multiview subspace clustering (rMV-spc) method. This was employed to discover common co-expressed genes, which can then be used as biomarkers for cancer stage prediction. protein-protein interaction (PPI) network was used as input an optimization was based on the interior point algorithm. This was applied to TCGA- Breast cancer dataset and was able to achieve satisfactory results.

A multiview spectral clustering method was employed by Yu and colleagues [35]for the clustering of multiview cancer data. Their optimization protocol involved the line search algorithm rather than eigenvector calculations. The method was applied to simulation and real data from TCGA and the performance was satisfactory.

In another study [36], Group Lasso regularised Deep learning (GDP) was applied to study cancer prognosis and survival prediction. This combines deep learning and Cox- Proportional Hazard model (CPH) on clinical and multi-omics data. They showed that the prediction accuracy was very high.

Thus it is seen that AI offers unique opportunities to understand and decode complex information generated from multi-omics data. AI algorithms have evolved specifically to address different aspects of biological data integration and prediction. The application of AI in this area of multiple data fields is limited by the availability of publicly available large curated datasets like TCGA. Meaningful extraction of clinical decisions will rely on future advances in sample extraction, clustering, and processing platforms.

AI IN DIGITAL IMAGING

Histopathology is a Science that deals with the study of disease status based on the cross-sectional view of tissue sections. It is a very old, yet reliable diagnostic technique for cancer. Even today, the majority of cancer grading and staging is done after careful histopathological examination. Very high accuracy in histopathology analysis is needed for personalized cancer therapy. Biomarker assessment in pathology slides especially requires a very good skill set in the pathologists. It is also limited by the fact that detecting the occurrence of biomarkers in a heterogeneous slide is challenging. Very recently, with the advancements in digital slide scanners, Whole Slide Images (WSI) has digitized the traditional slides [37]. This has envisioned a digital workflow for pathologists to improve their accuracy and precision in inappropriate decision making towards providing improvised patient care [38]. Computational pathology research initiatives have been geared up to improvise and speed up the assessment of morphological features and biomarkers in tissue sections [39].

Traditionally medical image analysis majorly relied on manual feature extraction, which was limited by the experts' knowledge in the specific area. With the exponential growth of WSI, this approach was not sufficient and lacked robustness and accuracy. Currently, deep learning is employed in solving tasks involved in image classification and categorization to an extent of surpassing manual performance.

Deep learning algorithms are also sought in this area, as the image data is tremendously large.Yet, computational pathology applications are not populardue to the limited availability of annotated image data sets. A small glass slide at 20 X magnification could produce files of several gigapixels. Also, this has led to the annotation of WSIs into a number of small tiles. This requires extensive annotations at the pixel level by pathology experts. Hence, this explains the relatively scarce availability of highly curated pathology datasets [40-43]. In a study by Ehteshami et al., [44], 399 WSIs were analyzed by deep convolutional neural networks. These outperformed pathology experts in breast cancer metastasis identification.

Campanella et al., [45] have developed a deep learning framework, combining convolutional neural networks with recurrent neural networks, under a Multiple Instance Learning (MIL) approach. This system has been applied to a large dataset of 732 WSIs from 15,187 patients. The analysis was performed without any manual data curation, across prostate, bladder and breast cancer metastasis. The authors were able to achieve 100% sensitivity, which could be deployed towards computational decision support by clinicians.

TCGA Image database has a collection of images from 25 anatomic sites ad 32 cancer subtypes. TCGA has a collection of 30,000 WSIs from approximately 11,000 patients and hence serves as the largest repository for training image datasets [46-48].

There are several deep learning tools employed in the annotation of WSIs and digital imaging initiatives.

The following table (Table 2) summarizes the utility of various neural network tools used in tumor image analysis.

Table 2. Neural network tools in tumor image informatics

Nature of the tool	Utility and Name	Reference
Supervised	Image classification (Convolutional Neural Networks CNN)	Wang et al.[49]
Feed Forward Network (FNN)	Image segmentation (FCN, Mask - RCNN)	He et al., [50]; Shelhamer et al. [51]
Recurrent Neural Network (RNN)	Multi label image classification (CNN- RNN) Image segmentation (Re Seg)	Wang et al. [42] Visin et al. [52]
Unsupervised	Auto – Encoder Image denoise Feature extraction Model pre training	Su et al. [53] Chang et al. [54]

Currently, supervised learning methods dominate biomedical and health applications. Supervised learning methods employ a training dataset with appropriate labels on them. Deep learning involves Artificial Neural

Networks (ANN). Deep learning models have various levels of hidden layers, for predicting an output for a given input. A typical CNN also has the above features. The hidden layers are composed of several convolutional features, which apply the same transformations at various positions of the image [43].

These layers are followed by several connected layers and these feed information to the output layer. A major advantage of CNN in image analysis is that it ensures end to end learning.

CNNs have been employed to detect breast cancer tubules [55]. Their study employed a deep learning classifier to automatically extract breast tubules from WSI of Estrogen Receptor positive breast cancer. Images containing the nuclei of cells were extracted and tubules were manually labeled. These were then used to train a DNN for tubule identification and its association with high and low-risk carcinomas.

In another study [56], the authors have utilized the potential of CNNs to stratify histopathology images of lungs into the normal lung, Lung Adeno Carcinoma (LUAD) and Lung Squamous Cell Carcinoma (LUSC). They initially classified the images as tumor or normal, followed by classification of tumors into LUAD or LUSC. The study used 163 WSI from GDC, which had 1176 tumor tissue samples and 459 normal samples. The slides were divided into training, validation and testing sets. The training was performed in a 512 X 512-pixel tiles and hence, tens to thousands of such tiles per slide were analyzed. They were able to achieve an accuracy of 96.1% per tile. Inception v3 architecture was trained with the training datasets. Back propagation, cross-entropy loss and RMSProp optimization methods were used for both training and test datasets. It has been shown that this CNN model outperformed manual identification of LUAD and LISC class.

Deep learning applications in cancer digital pathology imaging is not just limited to tumor grading and staging, but also attempts to investigate on several molecular features. Wang et al. [49], have predicted the recurrence rate in early stage non small cell lung cancer by extracting nuclear features from the Hematoxylin – Eosin (HE) images.

Kulkarni et al. have[57] predicted prognosis from HEimages of melanoma. They have used a deep neural network architecture to detect Disease Specific Survival (DSS) in early stage melanoma.

Survival rates were predicted in Glioma with the data from 1061 WSIs and correlated the data with TCGA patient survival data. In this study, CNN was integrated with Cox hazard model to predict patient outcomes [58].

Mostavi et al. [59] have use CNNs to predict cancer types from TCGA dataset using gene expression profiles. The authors were able to identify well known breast cancer markers like GATA3 and ESR1. They were also able to achieve 88.2% accuracy among 5 subtypes.

The above literature illustrates the role of AI in revolutionizing digital pathology. Although undoubtedly AI outperforms human interventions, there are few key limitations and challenges to be resolved with AI applications. The complexity with which AI models derive at the output is considered a 'black box' problem. Another major area of concern is the need to train AI models with a huge training set, which is not currently available, other than the TCIA. Nevertheless, AI incorporation is the next massive leap in the area of precision pathology.

CONCLUSION

Recent technologies have made the generation of Biological data cost effective and hence there is a data boom. Computational tools are sought for combining these multidimensional data and integrate them into meaningful clinical decisions. Especially cancer data is heterogeneous, with a small number of samples and a large number of measurements. There is also a large noise in the data. Hence, computational algorithms should be specifically modified to address these challenges, which are not usually seen in other types of big data. AI intervention in personalized cancer cure has a huge potential, which needs to be tapped. Given the tremendous increase in cancer research, clinical trial data, drug discovery modules, multi-omics information and imaging advancements, there is an emerging need for highly evolved AI tools in assisting towards biomarker identification and to guide in clinical decision making. Although an enormous increase is seen concerning the number of research articles published in the field of AI and cancer Biology, a lot of challenges are still in front to be solved. For a successful translation of computing tools from the lab to bedside, many of the knowledge gaps need to be addressed. Although many AI algorithms are available, a judicious selection of the algorithm for a specific application requires expertise. Informaticians have a limited knowledge of oncology set up and hence collaborative initiatives between clinical oncologists, research group and data scientists are the need of the hour to fully trap the potential of AI in cancer care and diagnostics.

REFERENCES

[1] Siegel, Rebecca L et al. 2020. "Cancer statistics, 2020." *CA: a cancer journal for clinicians* 70.

[2] Burrell, Rebecca A et al. 2013. "The causes and consequences of genetic heterogeneity in cancer evolution." *Nature* 501: 338-45.

[3] Chial, Heidi.2008. "DNA sequencing technologies key to the Human Genome Project." *Nature Education*1:219.

[4] Goodwin, Sara et al. 2016. "Coming of age: ten years of next-generation sequencing technologies." *Nature reviews. Genetics* 17: 333-51.

[5] Lowe, Rohan et al. 2017. "Transcriptomics technologies." *PLoS computational biology* 13: e1005457.

[6] Kukurba, Kimberly R, and Stephen B Montgomery. 2015. "RNA Sequencing and Analysis." *Cold Spring Harbor protocols* 11: 951-69.

[7] Tomczak, Katarzyna et al. 2015. "The Cancer Genome Atlas (TCGA): an immeasurable source of knowledge." *Contemporary oncology (Poznan, Poland)* 19: A68-77.

[8] Li, Yifeng et al. 2018. "Genome-wide prediction of cis-regulatory regions using supervised deep learning methods." *BMC Bioinformatics* 19: 202.

[9] Szymczak, Silke et al. 2009. "Machine learning in genome-wide association studies." *Genetic epidemiology* 33: S51-7. doi: 10.1002/gepi.20473.

[10] Telenti, Amalio et al. 2018. "Deep learning of genomic variation and regulatory network data." *Human molecular genetics* 27: R63-R71. doi: 10.1093/hmg/ddy115.

[11] Cancer Genome Atlas Network. 2012. "Comprehensive molecular portraits of human breast tumours." *Nature* 490: 61-70.

[12] Way, Gregory P et al. 2018. "Machine Learning Detects Pan-cancer Ras Pathway Activation in The Cancer Genome Atlas." *Cell reports* 23: 172-180.

[13] Zou, H, Hastie T. 2005. "Regularlization and variable selection via the elastic net". *J R Statist Soc B* 67:301–320.

[14] Rendleman, Michael.C. et al. 2019. "Machine learning with the TCGA-HNSC dataset: improving usability by addressing inconsistency, sparsity, and high-dimensionality." *BMC Bioinformatics*20: 339.

[15] Tranchevent, Léon-Charles et al. 2019. "A deep neural network approach to predicting clinical outcomes of neuroblastoma patients." *BMC medical genomics* 12: 178.

[16] Ma, Tianle, and Aidong Zhang. 2019. "Integrate multi-omics data with biological interaction networks using Multi-view Factorization AutoEncoder (MAE)." *BMC genomics* 20: 20.

[17] Shen, Ronglai et al. 2009. "Integrative clustering of multiple genomic data types using a joint latent variable model with application to breast and lung cancer subtype analysis." *Bioinformatics* 25: 2906-12.

[18] Wu, Dingming et al. 2015. "Fast dimension reduction and integrative clustering of multi-omics data using low-rank approximation: application to cancer molecular classification." *BMC Genomics* 16:1022.

[19] Hoadley, Katherine A et al. 2014. "Multiplatform analysis of 12 cancer types reveals molecular classification within and across tissues of origin." *Cell* 158: 929-944.

[20] Bruno, Eric and Marchand-Maillet S. 2009. "Multiview clustering: A late fusion approach using latent models categories and subject descriptors". *Proc. ACM SIGIR '09* NY ACM Press: 736 – 737.

[21] Nguyen, Tin et al. 2017. "A novel approach for data integration and disease subtyping." *Genome research* 27: 2025-2039.

[22] Wang, Bo et al. 2014. "Similarity network fusion for aggregating data types on a genomic scale." *Nature methods* 11: 333-7.

[23] Wang, Hua et al. 2013. "Multi-view clustering and feature learning via structured sparsity." in *Proc. ICML 13:* 352 – 360.

[24] Bickel, S and T. Scheffer. 2004. "Multi-view clustering", in *Proc. 4th IEEE Int. Conf. Data Mining*, Brighton, UK pp. 19–26.

[25] deSa Virginia, R. 2005. "Spectral Clustering with Two Views". In the *Proceedings of the Workshop on Learning with Multiple views, 22nd ICML 2005*;20 – 27.

[26] Kumar Abhishek et al. 2011. "Co-regularized multi-view spectral clustering." In *Proc. NIPS '11*.2011 USA. 1413 – 1421.

[27] ChikhiNasimFateh. 2018. "Multi-view clustering via spectral partitioning and local refinement". *Inform. Process. Manage.*52: 618 – 627.

[28] Li, Yeqinget al. 2015. "Large-scale multi-view spectral clustering with bipartite graph." In *Proc. AAAI 15*. 2750 – 2756.

[29] Wang, Shidan et al. 2019. "Pathology Image Analysis Using Segmentation Deep Learning Algorithms." *The American journal of pathology* 189: 1686-1698.

[30] Andrew, Galonet al.2013. "Deep canonical correlation analysis". *Proc. ICML 13*. 28:1247 – 1255.

[31] Chaudhary, Kumardeep et al. 2018. "Deep Learning-Based Multi-Omics Integration Robustly Predicts Survival in Liver Cancer." *Clinical cancer research: an official journal of the American Association for Cancer Research* 24: 1248-1259.

[32] Rappoport, Nimrod, and Ron Shamir. 2018. "Multi-omic and multi-view clustering algorithms: review and cancer benchmark." *Nucleic acids research* 46: 10546-10562.

[33] Yu, Yun et al. 2019. "Simultaneous clustering of multiview biomedical data using manifold optimization." *Bioinformatics (Oxford, England)* 35: 4029-4037.

[34] Zhang, Enli, and Xiaoke Ma. 2018. "Regularized Multi-View Subspace Clustering for Common Modules Across Cancer Stages." *Molecules (Basel, Switzerland)* 23: 1016.

[35] Yu, Na et al. 2018. "Co-differential Gene Selection and Clustering Based on Graph Regularized Multi-View NMF in Cancer Genomic Data." *Genes* 9:586.

[36] Xie, Gangcai et al. 2019. "Group Lasso Regularized Deep Learning for Cancer Prognosis from Multi-Omics and Clinical Features." *Genes* 10: 240.

[37] Fuchs, Thomas J, and Joachim M Buhmann. 2011. "Computational pathology: challenges and promises for tissue analysis." *Computerized medical imaging and graphics: The official journal of the Computerized Medical Imaging Society* 35: 515-30.

[38] Louis, David N et al. 2016. "Computational Pathology: A Path Ahead." *Archives of pathology & laboratory medicine* 140: 41-50.

[39] Colling, Richard et al. 2019. "Artificial intelligence in digital pathology: a roadmap to routine use in clinical practice." *The Journal of pathology* 249: 143-150.

[40] Valkonen, Mira et al. 2017. "Metastasis detection from whole slide images using local features and random forests." *Cytometry. Part A: the journal of the International Society for Analytical Cytology* 91: 555-565.

[41] Wang, Jiang et al. 2016. "CNN-RNN: A Unified Framework for Multi-label Image Classification." In *Proceedings of the 2016 IEEE*

Conference on Computer Vision and Pattern Recognition (CVPR), Las Vegas, NV, USA. 2285–2294.

[42] Janowczyk, Andrew and AnantMadabhushi. 2016. "Deep learning for digital pathology image analysis: A comprehensive tutorial with selected use cases." *Journal of pathology informatics* 7:29.

[43] Litjens, Geert et al. 2016. "Deep learning as a tool for increased accuracy and efficiency of histopathological diagnosis." *Scientific reports*. 6: 26286.

[44] EhteshamiBejnordi, Babak et al. 2018. "Using deep convolutional neural networks to identify and classify tumor-associated stroma in diagnostic breast biopsies." *Modern pathology: an official journal of the United States and Canadian Academy of Pathology, Inc* 31: 1502-1512.

[45] Campanella, Gabriele et al. 2019. "Clinical-grade computational pathology using weakly supervised deep learning on whole slide images." *Nature medicine* 25: 1301-1309.

[46] Prior, F, et al. 2013. "TCIA: an information resource to enable open science." In *Engineering in Medicine and Biology Society (EMBC), 2013 35th Annual International Conference of the IEEE*; 2013:. doi: 10.1109/EMBC.2013.6609742.

[47] Kalpathy-Cramer, Jayashree et al. 2014. "Quantitative Imaging Network: Data Sharing and Competitive Algorithm Validation Leveraging the Cancer Imaging Archive." *Translational oncology* 7: 147-52.

[48] Prior, Fred et al. 2017. "The public cancer radiologyimaging collections of The Cancer Imaging Archive." *Scientific data* 4: 170124.

[49] Wang, Xiang Xueet al. 2017. "Prediction of recurrence in early stage non-small cell lung cancer using computer extracted nuclear features from digital H&E images." *Scientific reports* 7: 13543.

[50] He, Kaiming et al. 2015. "Mask R-CNN." in *IEEE Int. Conf. Comp. Vis.* 2961–2969.

[51] Shelhamer, Evan et al. 2017. "Fully Convolutional Networks for Semantic Segmentation." *IEEE transactions on pattern analysis and machine intelligence* 39: 640-651.

[52] Visin, Francesco et al. 2016."ReSeg: A Recurrent Neural Network-based Model for Semantic Segmentation". *In Proceedings of the 2016 IEEE Conference on Computer Vision and Pattern Recognition Workshops (CVPRW),* Las Vegas, NV, USA, 426–433.

[53] Su, Hai et al. 2015. "Robust Cell Detection and Segmentation in Histopathological Images Using Sparse Reconstruction and Stacked DenoisingAutoencoders." *Medical image computing and computer-assisted intervention: MICCAI.International Conference on Medical Image Computing and Computer-Assisted Intervention* 9351: 383-390.

[54] Cheng, Jun et al. "2018. Identification of topological features in renal tumor microenvironment associated with patient survival." *Bioinformatics (Oxford, England)* 34: 1024-1030.

[55] Romo-Bucheli, David et al. 2016. "Automated Tubule Nuclei Quantification and Correlation with Oncotype DX risk categories in ER+ Breast Cancer Whole Slide Images." *Scientific reports* 6: 32706.

[56] Coudray, Nicolas et al. 2018. "Classification and mutation prediction from non-small cell lung cancer histopathology images using deep learning." *Nature medicine* 24: 1559-1567.

[57] Kulkarni, Prathamesh M et al. 2019. "Deep Learning Based on Standard H&E Images of Primary Melanoma Tumors Identifies Patients at Risk for Visceral Recurrence and Death." *Clinical cancer research: an official journal of the American Association for Cancer Research* 26: 1126-1134.

[58] Mobadersany, Pooya et al. 2018. "Predicting cancer outcomes from histology and genomics using convolutional networks." *Proceedings of the National Academy of Sciences of the United States of America* 115: E2970-E2979. doi:10.1073/pnas.1717139115.

[59] Mostavi, Chiuet al.2020. "Convolutional neural network models for cancer type prediction based on gene expression". *BMC Med Genomics* 13: 44.

In: Computing Paradigms for Smart Healthcare ISBN: 978-1-53618-619-2
Editors: B. Vinoth Kumar et al.

Chapter 8

DNA MICROARRAY TECHNOLOGY IN HEALTHCARE 4.0

S. Akila* and S. Allin Christe, PhD
Department of Electronics and Communication Engineering,
PSG College of Technology, Coimbatore, India

ABSTRACT

The steady progression in the healthcare technology has led to the Healthcare 4.0. The impact of the health care applications in the prognosis and diagnosis of diseases is significant. The technologies like virtual reality, Machine learning and deep learning plays a prominent role in the Healthcare 4.0. The DNA microarray technology being an upcoming area in the disease diagnosis and prognosis highly relies upon the two key technologies of healthcare: Deep learning and Machine Learning. The DNA microarray data with very high dimension and highly informative genes are used for classifying the disease causing genes. For the Micro array data to be processed more efficiently the Machine Learning and deep learning algorithms are used. This chapter begins with a very brief introduction to DNA microarray data followed by the

* Corresponding Author's E-mail: akilascs19@gmail.com.

implementation of machine learning algorithms to obtain the highly predictive genes for classification. Performance analysis of the bio-inspired algorithms along with Machine Learning for classifying the DNA microarray data is presented.

Keywords: DNA microarray, Gene selection, Classification, Microarray gene reduction, Cancer

INTRODUCTION

The extension of the automation and data exchange technologies like big data, wireless internet mediums, cloud computing, cryptography, content based image retrieval and augmented reality from industry 4.0 to healthcare domain is referred to as healthcare 4.0. This has a very high potential to virtualized and provide the healthcare related process as service to the stakeholders by the healthcare industry. This enables us to provide the personalised medicines. With the growing trend in healthcare, the development trends were named as healthcare versions ranging from 1.0 to 4.0. Healthcare 1.0 involved in the processes of analysing and structuring the germ theory, inventing the vaccination processes and sanitation. Development of big hospitals with professionalism and speciality care along with the growth of the pharmaceutical industry and antibiotics made thehealthcare 2.0. The healthcare 3.0 involved the process of evidence based diagnosis with computation and imaging. Now, the current era of healthcare 4.0 is the artificial intelligence based medical diagnosis and prognosis for precision medicine and telemedicine. The main aim of involving artificial intelligence in the process of diagnosis of the disease is to provide treatment in early stages and to increase the quality of medical aid. The main and most prominent area of medical diagnosis to find a disease at a very early stage is the DNA microarray analysis [1-6].

DNA microarray data is used for analysing the prominent genes that causes disease or disorder in the human. It is also used to classify the normal and abnormal genes present in the gene sequence. The DNA microarray data contains the samples and gene features. These gene features comprising the microarray data are high dimensional and highly informative in nature. With the influence of healthcare 4.0, artificial intelligence is used in the process of analysing DNA microarray data. The gene features present in the DNA microarray are of high dimension with less number of corresponding samples. Thus the curse of dimensionality is present [7-8]. The dimension of the gene features has a direct impact on the classification accuracy. As the dimension of the data increases, the possibility of irrelevant and redundant genes occurs. Thus reducing the accuracy and performance of the diagnosis system [9-11].

In this study, the focus is made on the cancer microarray data. Since the cancer is considered being the most deadly disease, the diagnosis and prognosis of cancer will help in providing the proper treatment and provide a high rate of recovery. Microarray analysis is widely used in the diagnosis of cancer and is believed to be accurate in diagnosis and classification [12]. Analysing a microarray would provide a better understanding in the genes related to the cancer that causes and is involved in causing cancer, which in turn would provide aid in developing new medicines and therapy techniques [13].

Artificial Intelligence methods are highly beneficial in classifying the genes and aid the pathologist in identifying the cancer causing genes. Traditional classification methods are poor in handling the microarray gene data. Hence, the advanced technologies like machine learning and deep learning are employed in the process of gene feature selection and classification.

The process involves finding the most predictive gene features using the classification model. This helps in improving the classification accuracy and reducing the computational complexity [14]. Many machine learning algorithms were employed along with gene selection techniques to analyse the gene expressions [15].

In this chapter, a brief overview of DNA microarray data and algorithms used for gene selection and classification is done.

The chapter is organised as the follwing section discussing the various gene selection and classification algorithms involved followed by the discussions and conclusion.

ALGORITHMS FOR CANCER MICROARRAY DATA GENE SELECTION AND CLASSIFICATION

Advancement in early classification of the cancer causing genes from the normal genes will help the healthcare 4.0 in early diagnosis and precision treatment of the deadly cancer disease. The reason for developing a more precision treatment is that the same therapy may show different responses for different types of cancers. Classification algorithms involving in real time data involve either binary or multiple class classification. The study focuses on the classification algorithms involving statistical approaches, classifiers based machine learning approaches, and filter and wrapper based approaches for machine learning and deep learning models. The DNA microarray datasets used in this chapter are obtained from the evaluation is with number of samples ranging from 60 to 253 while the gene feature sets are between 2000 and 15154 obtained from the open repositiory [16]. The dimensions of the datasets are presented in terms of dataset (samples, genes): Leukemia (72,7129), Lung (181,12533), Colon (60,2000) and Ovarian (253,15154).

Statistical Methods

Statistical methods were involved in the process of classifying the microarray data in the literature. The traditional statistical approaches involve the process of data collection quantification and analysis followed by drawing conclusions. Principal Component Analysis (PCA) based principal component accumulation methods which in a data mining approach has been used for the pre-process of gene feature selection and classification [17]. Association rule based classification models that were easily understood by the clinical researchers were used [18]. Rule based model with higher accuracy called Boolean Structure Table Configuration (BSTC) was used to perform the classification [19]. Correlation Feature Selection (CFS) based gene feature selection and classification were performed to rank the genes and filter them for efficient classification [20]. Using the redundancy and irrelevant genes present in the microarray dataset, the minimun Redundancy and Maximun Relevance (mRMR) based filters were used [21]. Also the process of feature selection for an efficient classification was done using the Fast correlation based Filter (FCBF) [22]. A relief based algorithm was used for selecting the features and improving the classification accuracy [23].

Machine Learning Based Classification Models

Using the machine learning algorithms, the machine is made to learn microarray data and is made to train in such a way that it could distinguish the normal and abnormal genes. Support Vector Machines (SVM) are considered to work well for high dimension data. SVM based microarray classification methods have been used widely to perform cancer classification in microarray data. By maximizing and minimizing the margin of the hyper planes, the high classification accuracy is achieved [24-27]. Naive bayes(NB) classification algorithm derived from the bayes theorem is used for the process of classification of microarray genes [28-29]. Artificial Neural Network based an algorithm that has a self training capacity which mimics the activities of neurons present in the human body is also used for microarray classification [30]. K Nearest Neighbour(KNN) based algorithm in which the unidentified data is accommodated to the nearest class is used in the process of microarray data classification [31, 32]. Random Forest (RF) and decision trees are also used in the process of classification of the machine learning data [33, 34].

Optimization Algorithms for Classification

An optimal feature selection problem is categorised as NP-hard problem. Hence heuristic nature inspired algorithms are more suitable. Evolutionary algorithms are used in the process of gene feature selection and classification. Genetic Algorithm (GA) is one among the most prominent algorithms used in the process of gene selection and classification [32, 33]. Particle Swarm Optimization (PSO) algorithms based on the swarm intelligence is used for microarray cancer classification [34]. Artificial Bee Colony (ABC) optimization for gene feature selection and classification is proposed [35]. A combined hybrid algorithm comprising genetic algorithm and bee colony algorithm as Genetic Bee Colony (GBC) algorithm is proposed [35]. Firefly optimization algorithm with recursion is proposed as R-firefly for gene selection and classification [36]. Flower pollination algorithms were used to optimize and classify the cancer microarray data [37]. Artificial bat based algorithms were proposed to obtain the optimal gene features for the process of classification [38].

Hybrid Models

The hybrid models comprise a filter and wrapper component. Wrapper based algorithms were developed by hybridizing the nature inspired optimization algorithms and classifiers to evaluate the predictive genes that are obtained. Here in hybrid models, the dataset is subjected to the first level of processing using a filter followed by a wrapper algorithm. Correlation Feature Selection based improved binary Particle Swarm Optimization (CFS - iBPSO) algorithm is used to find the predictive gene features from the microarray data [39]. The mRMR filter algorithm is combined with the Bat Algorithm (mRMR - BA) [40], Artificaial Bee Colony algorithm (mRMR - ABC) [41] and Genetic Algorithm (mRMR -

GA) [42] and implemented for obtaining the highly predictive genes from the microarray dataset and producing high classification accuracy.

ANALYSIS AND DISCUSSION

From the Tables 1-4, the classification accuracy and the number of gene features selected are tabulated. The methods involved in producing the results are statistical based methods, machine learning based classification models, optimization algorithms and wrapper based algorithms. Table 1 containing the statistical based methods show high classification accuracy while the number of gene features have not been reduced much. Next, the machine learning based classification algorithms whose results are shown in Table 2 shows acceptable classification accuracy with the same high number of gene features.

Table 1. Classification Accuracy and Predictive Gene features obtained using Statistical methods

Method	Leukemia	Lung	Colon	Ovarian
PCC	97.06(7129)	99.33(12533)	-	-
BSTC	82.53(866)	100(2175)	-	100(2769)
CFS	96.75(81)	-	-	-
mRMR	91.18(130	-	90(10)	100(16)
FCBF	100(51)	-	85.48(14)	99.91(30)

Table 2. Classification Accuracy and Predictive Gene features obtained using Machine learning based classification models

Method	Leukemia	Lung	Colon	Ovarian
SVM	65.28(7129)	89.93(12533)	64.52(2000)	86.95(15154)
RF	94.44(7129)	91.27(12533)	80.65(2000)	94.07(15154)

Table 3. Classification Accuracy and Predictive Gene features obtained using Optimization algorithms for classification

Method	Leukaemia	Lung	Colon	Ovarian
GA	100(6)	-	93.55(12)	-
PSO	100(572.4)	99.30(2778)	74.19(478.1)	94.07
ABC	95.83(20)	97.91(8)	95.16(20)	5074.7
GBC	100(4)	100(4)	98.38(10)	-

Table 4. Classification Accuracy and Predictive Gene features obtained using hybrid filter and wrapper based models

Method	Leukaemia	Lung	Colon	Ovarian
CFS-iBPSO	100(4.3)	100(10.6)	94.84(42)	100(33)
mRMR-BA	100(5.23)	-	93.12(8.13)	100(3.83)
mRMR-ABC	100(14)	100(14)	96.77(15)	94.41(57)
mRMR-GA	93.05(51)	95.83(62)	95.16(83)	-

While Table 3 contains the optimization algorithms that produced high classification accuracy with minimum number of gene features. Though, the optimization algorithms produced high classification accuracy, the quality of the gene feature obtained is not known.

The next is the wrapper based algorithm which is a combination of nature inspired algorithm with a classifier which evaluates the gene feature subset.

Thus the Table 4 shows the good classification accuracy with the minimum number of gene features of good quality.

CONCLUSION

Thus this chapter clearly shows the experimental analysis of microarray gene data selection and classification that plays a prominent role in Healthcare 4.0 involving in the diagnosis and prognosis of diseases. The experimental investigation of the various algorithms is carried out and their classification accuracy along with the reduced gene features is obtained.

From the experimental study it is found that the wrapper based algorithms involving the optimization algorithm along with a classifier to evaluate the obtained gene features is more powerful. Further, the study can be extended to deep learning based models for microarray gene selection and classification.

References

[1] Hermann, M., Pentek, T., Otto, B. 2015. *Design Principles for Industrie 4.0 Scenarios: A Literature Review.* Working Paper, Technical University of Dortmund.

[2] Spatz, E. S., Krumholz, H. M. and Moulton, B. W. 2017. Prime time for shared decision making. *JAMA,* 317(13):1309 - 1310, 2017 - 1310.

[3] López, B., Torrent-Fontbona, F., Viñas, R. and Fernández-Real, J. M. 2018. Single nucleotide polymorphism relevance learning with randomforests for type 2 diabetes risk prediction. *Artif. Intell. Med.,* 85:43 - 49.

[4] Dinesen, B., Nonnecke, B., Lindeman, D., Toft, E., Kidholm, K., Jethwani, K., Young, H. M., Spindler, H., Oestergaard, C. U., Southard, J. A., Gutierrez, M., Anderson, N., Albert, N. M., Han, J. J. and Nesbitt, T. 2016. Personalized Telehealth in the future: A global research agenda. *J. Med. Internet Res.,* 18(3): 53.

[5] Tuwatananurak, J. P., Zadeh, S., Xu, X., Vacanti, J. A., Fulton, W. R., Ehrenfeld, J. M. and Urman, R. D. 2019. Machine learning can improve estimation of surgical case duration: A pilot study. *J. Med. Syst.,* 43(3):44.

[6] The Lancet. 2018. Artificial intelligence in health care: within touching distance. *Lancet,* 390(10114):2739.

[7] Bayarri, M. Jesus, Berger, James O., Dawid, A. Philip and Heckerman, David. 2003. *Bayesian Factor Regression Models in the "Large p, Small n" Paradigm,* Bayesian Statistics 7 Oxford University Press, 723 - 732.

[8] Yao, B., Li, S. 2010. ANMM4CBR: A case-based reasoning method for gene expression data Classification, *Algorithms Mol. Biol.,* 5 (1).

[9] Wu, M.-Y., Dai, D.-Q., Shi, Y., Yan, H., Zhang, X.-F. 2012. Biomarker identification and cancer classification based on microarray data using Laplace Naive Bayes model with mean shrinkage, *IEEE/ACM Trans. Comput. Biol. Bioinform.,* 9 (6) 1649 - 1662, doi: 10.1109/TCBB.2012.105.

[10] Jain, A. and Zongker, D. 1997. Feature selection: Evaluation, application, and small sample performance, *IEEE transactions on pattern analysis and machine intelligence,* 19(2) 153 - 158. doi: 10. 1109/34.574797.

[11] Saeys, Y., Inza, I., Larra naga, P. 2007. A review of feature selection techniques in bioinformatics, *Bioinformatics,* 23 (19)2507 - 2517. doi: 10.1093/bioinformatics/btm344.

[12] Simon, R. 2009. Analysis of DNA microarray expression data. *Best Pract. Res. Clin. Haematol.,* 22 (2), 271 - 282.

[13] Alba, E., Garcia-Nieto, J., Jourdan, L., Talbi, E.-G. 2007. Gene selection in cancer clas- sification using PSO/SVM and GA/SVM hybrid algorithms. In: *IEEE Congress on Evolutionary Computation,* 2007 (CEC 2007), pp. 284 - 290.

[14] Javed Khan, Jun Wei. 2001. M.R.: Classification and diagnostic prediction of cancers using gene expression profiling and artificial neural networks. *Nature Medicine,* 7(6), 673 - 679.

[15] Alshamlan, H., Badr, G., Alohali, Y. 2014. A comparative study of cancer classification methods using microarray gene expression profile. In: *DaEng,* vol. 285 of Lecture Notes in Electrical Engineering. Springer, pp. 389 - 398.

[16] Zexuan Zhu, Ong, Y. S. and Dash, M. 2007. Markov Blanket-Embedded Genetic Algorithm for Gene Selection, *Pattern*

Recognition, 49 (11), 3236 - 3248, (link:http://csse.szu.edu.cn/staff/zhuzx/Datasets.html).

[17] Liu, J., Cai, W., Shao, X. 2011. Cancer classification based on microarray gene expression using a principal component accumulation method. *Science China Chemistry,* 54, 802 - 811 (2011).

[18] Wang, X., Gotoh, O. 2009. Microarray-based cancer prediction using soft computing approach. *Cancer Informatics*, 7, 123 - 139.

[19] Iwen, M., Lang, W., Patel, J. 2008. Scalable rule-based gene expression data classification. In: *Data Engineering, ICDE*, 2008. IEEE 24th International Conference. 1062 - 1071.

[20] Hall, M. A. 2000. Correlation-based feature selection for discrete and numeric class machine learning,' In: *Proc. Int. Conf. Mach. Learn.,* 359 - 366.

[21] Ding, C., Peng, H. 2005. Minimum redundancy feature selection from micro array gene expression data, *J. Bioinform. Comput. Biol.,* 3 (02) 185 - 205. doi: 10.1142/S0219720005001004.

[22] Yu, L., Liu, H. 2003 Feature selection for high-dimensional data: a fast correlation-based filter solution, *ICML,* 3 856 - 863.

[23] Wang, Y., Makedon, F. 2004. Application of relief-F feature filtering algorithm to selecting informative genes for cancer classification using microarray data, In: *IEEE Proceedings Computational Systems Bioinformatics Conference,* CSB2004, 497 - 498. doi: 10.1109/CSB.2004.1332474.

[24] Alba, E., Garcia-Nieto, J., Jourdan, L., Talbi, E. 2007. Gene selection in cancer classification using pso/svm and ga/svm hybrid algorithms. In: *IEEE Congress Evolutionary Computation CEC,* 2007. 284 - 290.

[25] Furey, T. S., Cristianini, N., Duffy, N., Bednarski, D. W., Schummer, M., Haussler, D. 2000. Support vector machine classification and validation of cancer tissue samples using microarray expression data, *Bioinformatics,* 16 (10) 906 - 914. doi: 10.1093/bioinformatics/16.10.906.

[26] Guyon, I., Weston, J., Barnhill, S. and Vapnik, V. 2002. Gene selection for cancer classification using support vector machines. *Machine Learning*, 46 389 - 422. doi: 10.1023/A:1012487302797.

[27] Ramaswamy, S., Tamayo, P., Rifkin, R., Mukherjee, S., Yeang, C.-H., Angelo, M., Ladd, C., Reich, M., Latulippe, E., Mesirov, J. P. et al. 2001. Multiclass cancer diagnosis using tumor gene expression signatures, *Proc. Natl. Acad. Sci. U. S. A.,* 98 (26) 15149 - 15154. doi: 10.1073/pnas.211566398.

[28] Friedman, N., Geiger, D. and Goldszmidt, M. 1997. Bayesian network classifiers. *Machine Learning,* 29 131 - 163 doi: 10.1023/A:1007465528199.

[29] Kelemen, A., Zhou, H., Lawhead, P., Liang, Y. 2003. Naive Bayesian classifier for microarray data, *IEEE Proceedings of the International Joint Conference on Neural Networks,* 2003, 3 1769 - 1773.

[30] Narayanan, A., Keedwell, E., Tatineni, S. S. and Gamalielsson, J. 2004. Artificial neural networks for gene expression analysis, *Neuro computing,* 61 217 - 240.

[31] Narendra, P. M., Fukunaga, K. 1977. F.K. 1977. A branch and bound algorithm for feature subset selection. *IEEE Trans. Comput.,* 26 (9) 917 - 922, doi: 10.1109/TC.1977.1674939.

[32] Li, L., Pedersen, L. G., Darden, T. A., Weinberg, C. R. 2002. Computational analysis of leukaemia microarray expression data using the GA/KNN method, In: *Methods of Microarray Data Analysis,* Springer, 81 - 95 doi: 10.1007/978-1-4615-0873-1_7.

[33] Paul, T. K. and Iba, H. 2005. Gene selection for classification of cancers using probabilistic model building genetic algorithm, *BioSystems,* 82 208 - 225 doi: 10.1016/j.biosystems.2005.07.003.

[34] Chen, K.-H., Wang, K.-J., Wang, K.-M., Angelia, M.-A. 2014. Applying particle swarm optimization-based decision tree classifier for cancer classification on gene expression data, *Appl. Soft Comput.,* 24 773 - 780. doi: 10.1016/j.asoc.2014.08.032.

[35] Alshamlana, Hala M., Badra, Ghada H., Alohalia, Yousef A. 2015. Genetic Bee Colony (GBC) algorithm: A new gene selection method

for microarray cancer classification, *Computational Biology and Chemistry,* 56 49 - 60 doi: 10.1016/j.compbiolchem.2015.03.001.

[36] Dif, Nassima, Elberrichi, Zakaria. 2019. An Enhanced Recursive Firefly Algorithm for Informative Gene Selection, *International Journal of Swarm Intelligence Research,* 10(2) doi: 10.4018/IJSIR. 2019040102.

[37] Muhammad Nasiru Dankolo, Nor Haizan Mohamed Radzi, Roselina Salehuddin, Noorfa Haszlinna Mustaffa, 2018. Hybrid flower pollination algorithm and support vector machine for breast cancer classification, *Journal of Technology Management and Business*, 5.

[38] Sashikala Mishraa, Kailash Shawb, Debahuti Mishra. 2012. A New Meta-heuristic Bat Inspired Classification Approach for Microarray Data, *Procedia Technology,* 4 802 - 806.

[39] Indu Jain, Vinod Kumar Jain, Renu Jain. 2018. Correlation feature selection based improved-Binary Particle Swarm Optimization for gene selection and cancer classification, *Applied Soft Computing*, 62 203 - 215. doi: 10.1016/j.asoc.2017.09.038.

[40] Alomari Osama Ahmad and Ahamad Tajudin Khader, Mohammed Azmi Al-Betar, Laith Mohammad Abualigah. 2017. Gene selection for cancer classification by combining minimum redundancy maximum relevancy and bat-inspired algorithm, *Int. J. Data Mining and Bioinformatics,* 19(1). doi: 10.1504/IJDMB.2017.

[41] Alshamlan, H., Badr, G. H., Al-Ohali, Y. 2015. mRMR-ABC: a hybrid gene selection algorithm for microarray cancer classification, *Bio. Med. Res. Int. J.,* 2015. doi: 10.1155/2015/604910.

[42] El Akadi, A., Amine, A., El Ouardighi, A. and Aboutajdine, D. 2011. A two-stage gene selection scheme utilizing MRMR filter and GA wrapper, *Knowledge and Information Systems,* 26 (3) 487 - 500. doi: 10.1007/s10115-010-0288-x.

In: Computing Paradigms for Smart Healthcare ISBN: 978-1-53618-619-2
Editors: B. Vinoth Kumar et al.

Chapter 9

ACCELERATING PATIENT RECORD RETRIEVAL IN BLOCKCHAIN BASED ELECTRONIC HEALTH RECORDS SYSTEM USING KEY-VALUE STORES

P. RM. Pitchappan**, R. Tarun Aravind and G. R. Karpagam

Department of Computer Science and Engineering,
PSG College of Technology, Coimbatore, Tamil Nadu, India

ABSTRACT

Blockchain is a distributed ledger network which can be used to store data. In Blockchain, since each node depends on the previous node the structure provides sequential access to users. Electronic health records (EHRs) are used in hospitals nowadays to provide ease of access for both patients and practitioners to relevant medical records. But due to the sensitive nature of the data, there are data security, integrity, and transparency concerns over the data handled. This can be solved by

* Corresponding Author's Email: pitchappanprm@gmail.com.

implementing a Blockchain based EHR system such that the data's security, integrity and transparency can be assured. Since Blockchain is a sequential access structure, the search requests and retrieval of patient data is inefficient. This chapter proposes various data structures such as hash tables and prefix-based search trees to efficiently query the EHR data present in the Blockchain. Radix Tree is a prefix-based search tree where the EHR data is stored in the form of a key-value pair, where the key is a unique identifier. Similarly, we also implement hash tables and also compare the performance between the two. We also have considered a more efficient variant of these structures based on the demand of the data. We also accelerate the entire process by enabling our structures to utilize the parallel cores of a GPU. The results show that implementation of Key-Value Stores can significantly improve the time to query transactions in a Blockchain even when implemented in a CPU. The usage of Radix Trees in an environment where CPU is used for hashing for GPU is used for EHR retrieval displays the best performance among the various architectural combinations tried.

Keywords: electronic health records, Blockchain, data structures, key-value store, GPU

INTRODUCTION

Technology is revolutionizing all aspects of our life. We once used to take a bunch of reports and prescriptions before going to the doctor nowadays all we need to do is just provide our identification at the hospital and all our health records pop up. Nowadays patient records are stored in the form of Electronic Health Records (EHR) and Electronic Medical Records (EMR) [14]. They are all stored in a system provided by the hospital where the patients are asked to trust them that their data won't be misused or tampered with and we still trust a third party with our data.

The currency we use is issued by banks which are essentially a third party in most scenarios. Thanks to the growing advances in technology, we can now opt for peer to peer electronic currency systems, also called cryptocurrency, which facilitates transfer of tokens, which translate to a concrete monetary value in the real world, between two parties without the involvement of any third parties. One might wonder who maintains the ledger and what if there is a security issue such as Byzantines Fault which is a common issue is decentralized systems. We employ consensus algorithms that validate each transaction and groups them into blocks and linking them with the previous blocks sequentially thus the name Blockchain. This technology also helps in verification the transactions. The electronic currency, Bitcoin, which introduced us to Blockchain uses a proof of work consensus algorithm [1] [5]. Some of the salient features of a Blockchain network are data integrity, security, and transparency.

Storing data as records is a good analogy to how transactions are stored in a distributed ledger. Hence Blockchain can be used in places where the integrity and the security of the data stored are of utmost importance [12].

Blockchain can be integrated into healthcare to store and maintain EHRs and EMRs. Once integrated the patients need not worry about their data being misused or tampered with because they are computationally infeasible to do so.

The Blockchain network will also face several queries for patient records. Conventionally Blockchain is a sequential structure with no random access. Thus, each query will have to search through records in a linear manner, taking a long time. This affects the productivity of the system on a good day and worse scenarios on a bad day because the main reason for maintaining a digital record is to have immediate access to the data whenever necessary.

In this chapter, we explore the usage of Key-Value stores and the possibilities of applying Graphics Processing Units to improve the speed of transaction retrieval in Blockchains. The results show that using KVS along with the existing Blockchain architecture can show a significant improvement in time compared to the default method of accessing the transactions [16].

This chapter is exploring the usage of KVS to speed up transaction retrieval in Blockchains and also provides an introduction to the underlying technologies and its implementation in EHR systems. The organization of the chapter is as follows

1. Introduction - In this section, a brief overview of this chapter, the problem statement, the proposed solution and the results are discussed.
2. Chapter Organization – This section describes how the chapter is structured and can serve as a quick reference guide to a specific topic
3. Literature Survey – This section is a study of journals and articles of work that has already been done in the field of research that this chapter is based on
4. Blockchain Technology – This section gives an overview of the basics of Blockchain technology and its functionality
5. EHR and Blockchain – This section gives an introduction to Electronic Health Records and how Blockchain can be used to improve them
6. Key Value Stores – this section deals with the explanation and implementation of KVS to help hasten HER record retrievals in Blockchain and also explores 4 different ways of implementing the same.
7. Performance Evaluation –This section illustrates how using KVS can show significant improvements in record retrieval by plotting graphs and establishing a baseline using the default Linked List search implementation
8. Conclusion and Future Work – This section gives a summary of the chapter and discusses possible avenues to further improve the methods proposed in this chapter
9. References – This section lists all research works and articles that were referred while authoring this chapter

LITERATURE SURVEY

Blockchain is a peer to peer electronic communication and data storage system which was initially used by Bitcoin which is a peer to peer electronic currency that enables the transfer of currency from one party to another without the involvement of any third party. The transactions cannot be reversed and they can be verified easily. The proof of work consensus algorithm enables the integrity and the security factors of the electronic currency. This was first introduced by Satoshi Nakamoto in his white paper "Bitcoin: A Peer-to-Peer Electronic Cash System" [1]. The proof of work consensus is a computationally demanding process, this is used to validate a block of transactional data in a Blockchain but this validated block can be easily verified. The performance of the validation task can be improved significantly. The research "Improving Blockchain Security Validation and Transaction Processing Through Heterogeneous Computing" - 2019 by Ciprian Pungila, and Viorel Negru proposes a heterogeneous architecture coupled with an efficient storage model for instant transfers of data between memory and video memory, the validation process efficiency can be improved and offloaded from the CPU, with a direct result in increased transactional speeds and enhanced security [11]. Here the procedure follows in a way that a classic Merkle tree is considered and it is serialized in such a way that it can be transferred between the RAM and VRAM in a single burst which in turn leads to an increase in the number of transactions. GPUs graphical processing unit consists of several cores when compared to a conventional processor unit. This is built on the SIMD architecture. It accelerates the processes running in a computer by taking over the computationally intensive tasks from the CPU and processing it in parallel. "A Systematic Review of Blockchain Hardware Acceleration Architectures" by O'Mahony, Aidan T Popovici, and Emanuel M reviews research work on hardware level acceleration for Blockchain and in them, GPU is a prominent method [13]. They have shown to improve almost all aspects of a Blockchain including but not limited to searching, hashing, mining, and validation of blocks. Blockchain, a distributed ledger, is used to store transactional data between two parties. This can be modified to be used for general recordkeeping purposes such that all of the Blockchain's salient features are implicit into the recordkeeping system.

The research work "Blockchain Technology and Recordkeeping" by Victoria L. Lemieux, Darra Hofman, Danielle Batista, and Alysha Joo deals with the merits and demerits of storing Electronic health records, bank statements, etc. the kind of data that must be stored in an immutable environment. It also deals with current ownership and legal aspects of storing records in Blockchain [12]. A patient's Electronic Health Record will be stored in the hospital's system for easy reference and also for future purposes. But there always lies an ambiguity regarding its integrity, security, and transparency. "Using Blockchain for Electronic Health Records" by Ayesha Shahnaz, Dr. Usman Qamar, and Dr. Ayesha Khalid discusses the possibility and provides a system design for integrating Blockchain to store EHR. The design also involves a distributed adaptive file system to facilitate smart contracts. The EHR data can be stored in the form of a key-value pair considering a unique identifier as the key [14]. Blockchain uses a Merkle tree to verify the validity of a block using its hash but the block's data is stored using a list. A list is a sequential access data structure, here it is designed such that the current block depends on the previous node. Thus, querying a Blockchain for a particular record is not an efficient process.

As Blockchain facilitates the storage of key-value pairs the usage of GPU accelerated prefix-based trees to improve the query performance of a Blockchain has been dealt in "Accelerating Blockchain Search of Full Nodes Using GPUs" by Shin Morishoma, and Hiroki Matsutani [10]. The performance is improved exponentially when the provided structure is implemented for querying the data. Storing EHR in a Blockchain network means that there will be users continuously querying the records based on a preset identifier. The Blockchain's naive approach to responding to the queries is computationally infeasible for the given scenario as time is pertinent there. This chapter deals with the process of accelerating the query process for EHR data stored in a Blockchain network keeping various computational architectures under consideration.

Blockchain Technology

Blockchain was first introduced by Satoshi Nakamoto as the backbone for his paper on digital cryptocurrency, i.e., Bitcoin [1]. While Nakamoto mainly used the technology to create a decentralized ledger for financial transactions which could safeguard against problems such as record falsification and double spending, it was soon adapted to be used in various other applications including but not limited to healthcare, secure communications and smart contracts [5].

Blockchain can be visualized as a chain of connected blocks that keeps growing as the number of transactions increase. Even though it is a single connected chain virtually, in the real world, it is completely decentralized. The data is spread among many devices called nodes and there are usually many copies of the same data. A group of nodes or a single node containing at least one copy of all data in a Blockchain is called a full node.

Each Block holds a batch of transactions which are secured using cryptographic hashing to provide data integrity and managed by peer-to-peer networks. Advantages of Blockchain include security, anonymity and integrity of data with absolutely no third-party intervention. These features make it an ideal technology to store data like Electronic Health Records and Legal Contracts [12] [14].

Blockchain Architecture

Each Blockchain begins with an initial block (also called the Genesis block) and then transactions group together to form new blocks which are then appended to the main chain. When a new transaction is made, the P2P network decides to create a new block. The new transaction is retrieved from the transaction pool, a pool of all transactions waiting to be created into a block and added to the Blockchain, and placed inside a block which is then broadcasted to all nodes in the network. Each node has their own full copy of a Blockchain and are called full nodes. Now, a node 'mines' to find a nonce value to prove that the data is valid and broadcasts it's result to all other nodes which then easily verify the data before growing the chain by appending the block [1][5]. The structure of a Blockchain is clearly depicted in Figure 1.

This process of adding a block to grow the Blockchain is done by nodes reaching a consensus about which blocks and transactions are valid and which are not. This validation is performed using mathematically tough to compute but easy to verify algorithms called Consensus Algorithms. When a node successfully performs a validation of a block, that node is rewarded with crypto-currency. This process of validating the transaction is known as mining and the node performing this validation is known as a miner. Once the validation is done, the block is added to the Blockchain. Only after this is a transaction considered complete.

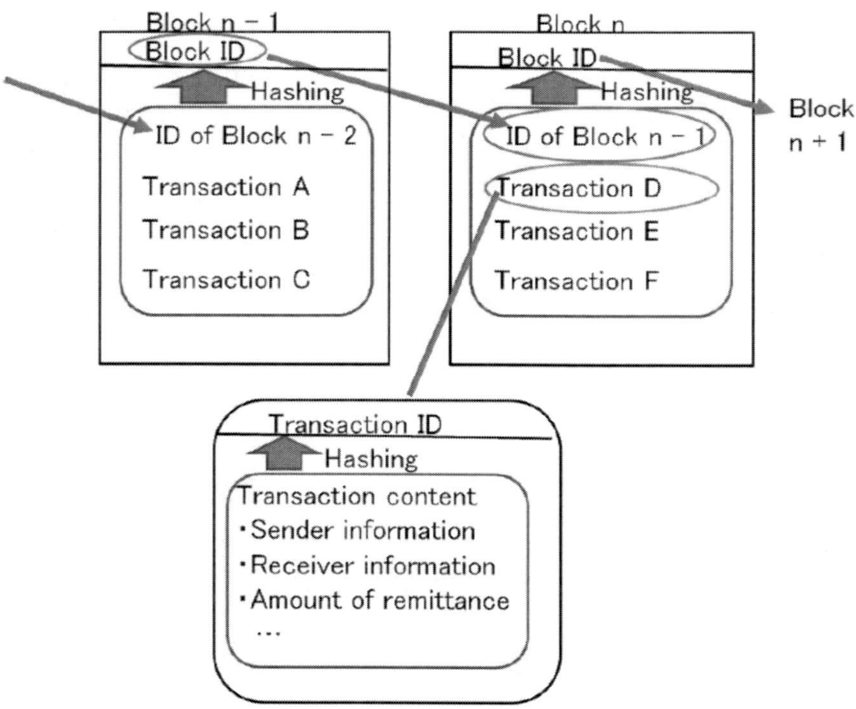

Figure 1. Overview of data structure of Blockchain.

BLOCK IN A BLOCKCHAIN

Figure 1 provides a clear depiction of a Blockchain and the role of Blocks. As shown in the top section of the diagram, Blockchain is a series of many blocks chained together, each of which contains details on the immediately previous block using previous block ID. A block ID is generated using the hashed value of data and thus affects all successive blocks, thus maintaining data integrity as a change in a single block will require a change in every single successive block. A block may contain multiple transactions and each transaction has a transaction ID and transaction contents [1].

As shown in the bottom half of the picture in Figure 1, The transaction ID is a hashed value of transaction contents and thus a change in the transaction is also protected against change of any form as it will change the hash value of the transaction, which will in turn change the value of the block's hash value and thus require a change in all successive blocks. A write query in the Blockchain only appends at the end and no updation or deletion is ever done.

Each Block has an upper limit for the data it contains, in the case Nakamoto's Bitcoin, the limit was 1 megabyte per block.

CONSENSUS ALGORITHMS

Whenever a block is added to the chain, it needs to follow some consensus rules to be valid for growing the Blockchain. For this purpose, Blockchains use complex mathematical operations to find a difficult to compute but easy to verify solution to a problem. Algorithms that facilitate this are called Consensus algorithms. The nodes that participate in the process of solving the problem are called miners and on providing a successful solution that leads to the addition of the block to the Blockchain, the miner receives a reward, usually in that Blockchain's native cryptocurrency. The most common consensus algorithm is the PoW

(Proof of Work) Algorithm used by Nakamoto for Bitcoin [1]. It involves guessing a nonce value for a block such that the SHA256 hash value of the total block matches a specified format. Other consensus algorithms include PoS (Proof of Stake), PoB (Proof of Burn), PoET (Proof of Elapsed Time), etc. [5].

FEATURES OF A BLOCKCHAIN

Decentralized

They are completely decentralized, meaning they answer to no central figure. They are run by a collective of nodes which prevent any one node from asserting control over the network.

Transparent

Blockchains consist of Blocks, and each block contains a number of transactions. Anyone with an access to a node can send a query across the network to verify the integrity of any transaction.

Immutable

In a Blockchain network the hash of each block depends on that of its predecessor, so in a Blockchain network tampering with the contents of a block means breaking the chain, which in turn leads to a smaller chain than the original one and it gets dropped.

Secure

The very implementation of Blockchain technology ensures security with mathematical certainty, making it almost impossible to change or destroy any record in the network. If someone did compromise the security of one particular node and edit the data, this change would be invalidated and overwritten with the original content by the other nodes.

Consensus Driven

Blockchains are consensus driven, meaning any and all changes will need the approval of at least 51% of the users ensuring a democratic element in the technology

SEARCHING IN A BLOCKCHAIN

Searching in a Blockchain for a particular transaction can be done in only a full node. The search is based on a doubly linked list where when you are in a block, you can either progress to the next block or backtrack to the previous block using the hash values [1]. When searching for a transaction, we usually begin at the genesis block (1st block in the chain) and then go forwards till we find the transaction we are looking for. The issue with this simple yet safe structure is the long time it takes to traverse a linked list to find details of transactions which might be a disadvantage when Blockchain is being integrated in applications where time is of the essence. This chapter aims to explore the usage of Key Value Stores to speed up searching time for transactions in a Blockchain and the possibility of using GPUs to speed up the same [2].

ELECTRONIC HEALTH RECORDS AND BLOCKCHAIN

An EHR (Electronic Health Records) is a digitized version of the traditional patient health chart and history file. EHRs are patient centered records that can make medical history and diagnostics instantly available to doctors and other authorized users in a secure manner in real time. Though they mainly contain medical histories of patients, they provide a more comprehensive and a customizable view of a patient's care.

One of the key and fundamental properties of Electronic Health Records is that the medical data can be created, managed and shared between numerous authorized providers across multiple healthcare organizations. EHRs share all types of information about a patient with many healthcare providers and organizations such as specialists, scanning facilities, hospitals, clinics, pharmacies, critical care units and schools and this facilitates EHRs to contain a comprehensive report from all professionals involved in a patient's care.

EHRs provide consistent and up-to-date medical information on all patients making it one of the next revolutionary changes in the healthcare industry. While using EHRs, guaranteeing the data integrity and security of the data is very important and Blockchain is one technology which is very apt for this application.

The E-healthcare system is believed to be one of the fields where Blockchain has great potential due to its inherent characteristics, especially for the management of electronic health records. Significant research efforts have been made in this direction in the last few years. Azaria et al., in 2016, put forth the idea for a decentralized HER system and coined it MedRec. The whole system was built on the Ethereum platform and used the Smart Contracts capability of the second generation Blockchain to create a representation of all available health records within all nodes in a network. MedRec allowed patients to control their personal records across healthcare providers inside the system. This also encouraged stakeholders in the medical services to participate in mining operations to keep the system functioning. The MedRec distributed Blockchain ledger maintains a detailed history of all documented medical interactions between patients and providers. This proposed solution raised an important question about how much control a patient should have over his own medical records. The related legislations have been redefined many times over the past decade and the grey areas are often dealt with by taking a path in accordance with the Hippocrates oath. For this reason, the available variation of the system should also be taken into the consideration that patients have not full control over their medical records and data are shared at different levels among all medical stakeholders [9].

While the storage of data and most other functionalities work well when storing EHRs in a Blockchain and using them with the default functions available in a Blockchain, Searching is one area where there is huge room for improvement. As discussed earlier in this chapter, Blockchain usually searches using a doubly linked list which can be improved using an intermediate data structure. This chapter proposes using a Key-Value Store methodology which is discussed in the next heading to store the data and explores storing the KVS in Radix trees and Hash tables and compares them with the default Linked List implementation.

Key Value Stores

A key-value store, or key-value database is a simple database that uses an associative array (think of a map or dictionary) as the fundamental data model where each key is associated with one and only one value in a collection. This relationship is referred to as a key-value pair.

In each key-value pair, the key is a unique identifier with each key pointing to one value, in this chapter's case, the virtual value. The value can be any kind of data. The value requires no schema definition as KVS in itself is this efficient mostly because of its simplicity. However, you cannot control or filter what's returned from a request because the value is of an opaque nature [16].

In general, key-value stores have no specific language or methodology for querying. They provide a way to store, retrieve and update data using simple GET, PUT and DELETE commands; the path to retrieve data is a direct request to the object in memory or on disk. This particular storage model is so simplistic that the storage and retrieval queries are fast, simplistic. The structure does not have much overheard so it can be easily scaled up. Partitioning (involves replication and auto recovery) is a technique using which these structures can be scaled. Some of the merits of this structure are that the entire DB can be maintained in the RAM which increases throughput and also the effects of acid are minimized by avoiding latches and low-overhead calls.

KVS Implementation in Blockchain

Blockchain search queries typically request transaction contents. KVS can be used for such queries given that the transaction address or some other unique id is assigned as a key and the corresponding data being the value. For Electronic Health Records, the patient's unique identifier (perhaps that is like a government issued citizenship ID) such as an Aadhar Card in India or one's Social Security Number in the United States of America can be the key and the corresponding value can point to the specific medical reports. Key-Value Store is uniquely suited for Blockchain in another way that there are no updations or deletions in a Blockchain. Harnessing this feature makes implementation of a KVS system more efficient for Blockchain search.

Keys and Values together make up Key-Value pairs. The GPU holds the keys and the CPU host memory contains the values. An index number is assigned to each value and this index value, which shall also be referred to as "virtual value" in this chapter is paired together with the keys and stored in the GPU. A pointer array in the CPU holds a mapping between the virtual value and the corresponding data. The virtual value of the first Key-Value pair is 0 and is incremented by 1 every time a new transaction is recorded. This system does not need to consider situations when a virtual value in the middle has no data because there can never be any form of modification in a Blockchain. Moreover, the Blockchain can be grown only at the last block, due to it being append only. Do note that the virtual value 0 corresponds to NULL which means the transactions in the genesis block begin at virtual value 1 for indexing.

In the GPU, a search query searches for a given key in all the existing keys in the GPU device memory and returns the corresponding virtual value. This virtual value can then be used to retrieve the actual data in the host CPU. In this method, the CPU-GPU transfer is very small, just a single virtual value. To accelerate the key search, we can store the KVS in the GPU in many ways [2].

The KVS search could be designed in many different structures and this chapter proposes a few different methods, the first 2 shall be implemented and the others are discussed theoretically

- Radix Tree
- Hash Table
- Modified Hash Table with Patricia Tree based chaining
- Adaptive Radix Tree

RADIX TREE

Trie and Radix trees (compressed Trie) provide means for an efficient key-value store. A trie (as in retrieval, re-trie-val) is a type of tree-based key-value store. The keys are a sequence of elements from some fixed alphabet, for example, strings. A key property of TRIE is that all the children/descendants of a node will share a common prefix in their keys. This means to all insertions and searching operations will execute with a complexity of O(k) where k is the bit length of the structures key. For easy understanding and simplicity, we choose arbitrary key-value pairs but actually, the key will be a unique identifier and the value segment holds the data. The steps involved in utilizing this structure are,

- Create an empty Trie. The root node is NULL
- Insert the pair ('AABBC', 1). Each letter gets a node, and the leaf node contains the value 1.
- Insert the pair ('XYZ', 2). There is no shared prefix, so the new data branches after the root. Similar to the previous key.
- Insert the pair ('ABX', 3). This shares a prefix with the already existing node 'AABBC'. So, this is added as a child to that node.
- Insert the pair ('XYZZ', 4). This also shares a prefix with the already existing node 'XYZ'. So, this is also added as a child.

```
Algorithm 1
Proposed Key Search on Radix Tree
1. V = 0 # current vertex
2. Search = 0 # digit of key currently being examined
3. P<0>[], P<1>[] # 1st and 3rd arrays
4. C<0>[], C<1>[] # 2nd and 4th arrays
5. Len # Key's bit length
6. Key[] # Bit pattern of key
7. While Search < Len:
     a. Temp = Search
     b. Search = Search + C<Key[Temp]>[V]
     c. V = P<Key[Temp]><Vr>
8. End while
9. Return V # virtual value of key
```

Figure 2. Algorithm for search in Radix Tree.

Formally when we consider insertion, we shall consider the below cases,

- Empty trie so create an empty node and insert here,
- There is no remaining key so add the value to the current node,
- Otherwise descend to the appropriate child and continue.

When performing search, we shall consider 3 cases,

- Empty trie so return no data,
- There is no remaining key to search so return the data at the current node,
- Otherwise descend to the appropriate child and continue searching with a shortened key.

When we consider the time complexity using trie the time required to find a key of length M is O(M) whereas in the case of other search trees the logarithmic value of the height is also taken into consideration. The simple trie implementation provided above suffers from at least one glaring issue; memory usage. If a single node leads to K references and the trie consists of N such identical nodes, then space complexity can be easily calculated as O(N*K). This also accounts for the fact that Null points also do occupy space. Whether an array entry is null or any other value doesn't change anything in terms of memory consumption.

The proposed algorithm for searching in a Radix tree is given in Figure 2

This can be solved by trading some time efficiency for space efficiency by replacing the slice of prefix nodes with a hashmap or a list (prefix, node) of pairs. But even after doing so a long key with no shared prefix will require each value in the key to be represented by a unique node. Here the naivest solution is the right one that is to compress the trie by merging nodes that have only one child. Now only the branch points need to allocate memory for children, and a long sequence of key data can be stored optimally. The radix tree will see its largest benefit when there are long prefixes of keys without any branches.

Here, the applications are similar to that of Trie but here the space-time trade-off is properly optimized such that higher efficiency can be achieved.

The implementation of the Radix Tree is fairly complex when compared with Tries. Here the node structure from Trie can be used with the addition of a second layer of pointers.

Insert procedure,

1. The radix tree is empty
   (a) The key is empty; insert a value node,
   (b) Insert a short Node with the key, call insert on the child.
2. The node contains Value
   (a) The key is empty; replace the value,
   (b) Create a branch with the existing data as a child, call insert on the branch.
3. The node is a FullNode
   (a) The key is empty; insert on the value child,
   (b) Call insert on the appropriate child node.
4. The node is a short Node
   (a) The shortNode. Key is a prefix of the key; call insert on the child,
   (b) There is no shared prefix of the keys; create a branch and insert short nodes child and the new (key, value) pair on the branch,
   (c) Create a branch as above, but insert it under a shortNode containing the shared prefix.

Explanation of terms used,

ValueNode - This node is used to store the value corresponding to a key. Its key field is empty.

FullNode - This is responsible for the reduction of the number of null children. This node holds the pointers that connect the shortNode and the valueNode.

ShortNode - This is responsible for handling the corresponding key substring based on its key prefix.

It can be seen that both Trie and Radix trees provide the same functionality one might ask the significance of Radix Trees. To provide the same functionality Tries uses over 4 times as much memory and performs at half the speed. This inference is based on the analysis performed on various benchmarks. Radix trees can be further improved by using adaptive nodes where the number of pointers of a node changes based on the number of child nodes. But in this chapter, we have considered plain binary radix trees.

HASH TABLE

One of the data structures we consider for storing our key-value pairs is the hash table. It is a data structure that stores data in an associative manner. Here the data is stored as an array, in an array each data can be accessed with its index (as array allows random access). Once the index is known the data can be accessed in constant time. Hash table is a structure that irrespective of data size permits constant access time to any random data stored in its structure. It also uses an array as a storage medium and the index is generated using the hash technique where the element can be inserted to or read from.

Each location in the table is referred to as a bucket. Inside each one of these buckets is a linked list containing the values of a key-value pair [6].

To insert data into the table, we need to process the key accordingly so that data can be placed in the right bucket. To do this we utilize a hash function that converts the key into a unique index which can then be used to find the respective bucket where the value shall be placed. From the unique index generated the bucket can be identified using the mod function which determines the bucket by keeping the size of the table into account. Based on the application, different hash functions can be implemented. Certain properties define a good hash function such that the output of a hash function must be unique for a given input, the size of the output must be the same irrespective of the input size and it must be computationally infeasible to reverse the function.

Once we have the hashed value of our key, we are ready to place our value into the corresponding bucket. The value returned from the hashing function is the index of the bucket that will hold our data. But with smaller table sizes, we will invariably reach a point when a new key also hashes to an already occupied row. This is called a collision. A collision is when more than one value is assigned to the same bucket, and this is a pretty common occurrence. There are several collision resolution techniques such as open addressing, chaining, and so on. The most basic yet effective method is called chaining. Here, the hashed result of the key does not point to the corresponding value. Instead, the hash key index acts as an intermediary to point us to an alternate data structure which holds multiple data points that were hashed into the same key. Linked lists is the most used data structure for chaining. Based on the application, table size and the hash algorithm the data structure used can be modified. In situations where collisions have high probability and it is a search application then instead of a linked list can use a search tree.

The proposed algorithm for searching in a hash table is given in Figure 3.

Algorithm 2
Proposed Search On Hash Table

```
1. Key[] # key to find value for
2. B[] # Buckets for hash table pointing to linked list
3. L[] # a linked list for each bucket
4. X # hash result
5. X = H(Key) # H(x) is the hash function
6. Not_found = 1 # bool value for not found
7. Ptr = L[B[X]]
8. If Ptr.key <> Key and Ptr.next <> NULL:
      a. Ptr = Ptr.next
      b. Not_found = 0
9. If Not_found == 1:
      a. Throw "not found"
10. Else:
      a. Return Ptr.value
```

Figure 3. Algorithm for search in Hash Table.

ADAPTIVE RADIX TREE

Radix trees are an improvement over the naive key-based search tree TRIE but it can be seen that during the implementation of radix trees not all of our pointers (based on the key) are used, this leads to wastage of space. The wasted space is not just a bad use of memory - which is in and of itself less and less concerning nowadays - but has real performance consequences in terms of the number of nodes that can be held. Bringing it under control is the key to ART (adaptive radix tree), and unlocks its biggest performance gains. The biggest change that Adaptive Radix Trees bring is the ability to dynamically change the data structure of each node using information such as how many children a node currently has, instead of the naïve method of basing the structure on how many it might have. As the number of children in a node changes, ART swaps out one implementation of the node structure for another. The paper distinguishes four different cases, for nodes with up to 4, 16, 48, and 256 children respectively [4].

Let us consider adaptive radix trees in detail now. From a complexity and performance point of view for radix trees, we need to find the sweet point of the right key size and span such that both space and time complexity is optimal. This the size of our nodes must change dynamically for every entry. But it is costly to modify the node size on the go. This is the inception of adaptive radix trees. We know that ART (adaptive radix tree) provides four different node sizes for its internal nodes. The general structure of the tree is the same as a regular radix tree. The node sizes were designed keeping the register sizes in various computer organizational architectures in mind. The structure as explained in the text is explained in Figure 4.

Node4 is the entry-level node. This is the smallest node that can store up to four keys. It also has another four-character array to store the corresponding pointers to the keys. A basic implementation would resemble,

Adaptive Radix Tree Structure

```
struct Node4
{
   char keys[4];
   Node* pointers[4];
}

struct Node16
{
   char keys[16];
   Node* pointers[16];
}

struct Node48
{
   char pointer_indexes[256];
   Node* pointers[48];
   char num_descendants;
}
   //to find a child key --
//->pointers[pointer_indexes[**key**] ]

struct Node256
{
      Node* pointers[256];
}

union Node
{
   Node4* N4;
   Node16* N16;
   Node48* N48;
   Node256* N256;
}
```

Figure 4. Structure of Adaptive Radix Tree.

Node16 is the node that is used to store between 5 and 16 keys. This functions similarly to the previous node structure. Here we use two 16 index arrays to store both the keys and pointers.

Both Node4 and Node16 searches a key using binary search or parallel comparisons in case of SIMD architecture.

Node48, we know that as the number of keys in a particular node increases the search process becomes costly and if we use the same technique as in the previous nodes a search would take around 384bits which cannot even be stored in a 256bit SIMD register.

So here we store the keys in a 256-index array. Here a separate 48 index array is used to point to the pointers. This is better as we can store 48 keys with 640 bytes itself. Here we will perform 2 offset calculations (data indirection) instead of 48 selections.

Node256 is the largest node structure. This simply stores 256 pointers. Here a single lookup is sufficient to find a key. No additional indirection is necessary.

The usage of these node structures depends on the usage and they are selected incrementally from lowest to highest.

It has been evaluated several times since the paper has been published, and is still considered an extremely competitive index implementation. It's appealing not only for its performance but for the minimal delta from a well-understood data structure that it represents.

Modified Hash Table with Patricia Tree Based Chaining

During the design phase of a hash table data structure, the designer chooses the hashing algorithm, the size, and other parameters of the structure based on the performance expected by the application, also factoring in the limitations such as collisions, scalability issues and so on. In hash tables, collisions are one of the most common issues. For handling collisions, we employ certain measures in the design phase itself. Chaining is one such strategy where the value is stored in a data structure that is present in the bucket so that when a collision occurs it can be handled. The go-to data structure is the linked list but it is not suitable in circumstances where a large number of key-value pairs collide.

Using a search tree in place of the linked list employs a logarithmic time search within the search but if we employ a radix/Patricia tree in place the search times can be improved drastically in case several collisions occur. All the functionalities of a radix tree will be present in every bucket of the table, within which the values are arranged based on the keys and the search complexity depends on the size of the key. The functioning is the same as explained in the previous topics.

Performance Evaluation

We compare the insertion and querying performance of the structures discussed in the previous sections against the naive Blockchain approach for EHR data structured to be a key-value pair,

1. Radix Tree
2. Hash Table

3. Linked List

A workstation grade computer with 16GB memory 4-core Intel-i7 running at 3.6 GHZ. The EHR data was generated randomly based on the format extracted from a dataset published online by California Health and Human Services [17]. GPU used was a single NVidia GTX1060 6GB VRAM, memory speed 8 Gbps, a clock speed of 1708 MHz with a boost of 1.4x with 1280 CUDA enabled cores.

The performance between the structures has been compared in Figure 5 and Figure 6.

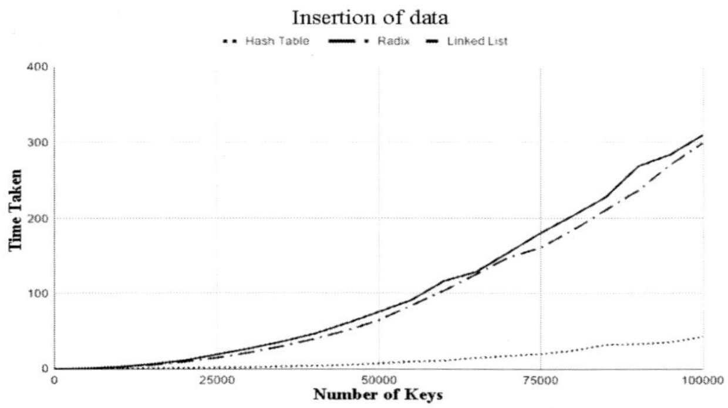

Figure 5. Relationship between number of keys to insert and time in seconds for Hash Table, Linked list and Radix Tree.

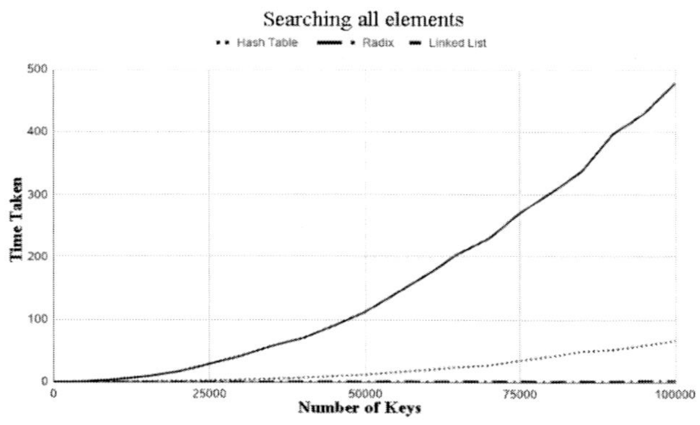

Figure 6. Relationship between number of keys and time to search all the keys in a hash table, Radix tree and Linked list.

Figure 5 compares the insertion time 100000 key-value pairs of randomly generated EHR data as explained before. Here it can be seen that the Hash table has a near-constant insertion time whereas the time taken for Linked List and radix trees increases with an increase in the number of keys. The time is taken by hash table also begins to increase towards the end, this is due to collision. Figure 6 compares the search time for all the keys that were inserted into the respective structures. The time taken by Linked List increases near linearly with an increase in the number of keys to be searched. Hash Table has a near-constant access time but towards the end, the time is taken increases due to collision of the keys, due to which we have to sequentially traverse the buckets for a particular index. Here for searching, it can be seen that the radix tree has the best performance. But the same cannot be told for the overall performance of the structure. So, it is safe to assume that a combination of these structures shall be used for the application. The exact combination shall be designed based on the data type (here we use text-based data), size, and various other factors.

General Purpose Graphics Processing Units (GPUs) have been used in many applications and fields in recent years to significantly increase efficiency and speed of computing in domains where the problem can be vectorized into subcomponents that can be executed parallelly. Contrary to CPUs, GPUs can handle many thousands of parallel threads, allowing for a great increase in the parallel processing of data. This increase has led to improving the performance of many applications, as significant speedups can be achieved by using optimized algorithms and lock-free data structures. Not many hash tables are optimized to utilize the parallelism provided by GPUs. Cuckoo hashing-based lookup tables can be used with GPUs to achieve an exponential increase in throughput. Alcantra et al. demonstrated a data-parallel algorithm for building hash tables on the GPU. It is available as part of CUDPP [7] [8] [15].

Performance measured using a GTX1060 CUDA enabled GPU card, inserts 64 million randomly generated EHR key-value pairs in 210 milliseconds, and deletes 32 million of those key/value pairs in about 64 milliseconds. Here a fixed-size hash table was used and the hash table must be of the size to the power of two.

The steps involved in increasing the size of the hash table is creating a new hash table of larger size and refilling the new table with the key-value pairs accordingly.

In a radix tree, a single thread is enough to match a key and return its value. In radix trees using GPUs to process the queries enables the system to process several queries in parallel which is not possible in a serial processing system. Introducing GPUs facilitates the system to scale easily, as mentioned earlier the keys are stored in the GPU memory where they are stored in a vectorized form and the corresponding values are stored in CPU memory [3]. The size and number of nodes of the tree depend on the size of the key (identifier) used. This condition is the same for both CPU based and GPU based systems. The memory usage is directly proportional to the number of keys. To achieve a greater throughput GPU avoids accessing the main memory which is relatively slower, it stores the entire data that is required in its dynamic memory such that the access latency is reduced and a greater throughput can be achieved. This is why a combination of CPU and GPU is used to achieve the desired performance efficiently.

For 3*10^20 keys a GPU only system uses 1.4GB whereas a combination of CPU and GPU uses 500MB only. When compared over a range it can be seen that CPU+GPU uses only a third of the keys used by GPU. The above recordings are from randomly generated EHR with text-based records only. In a CPU only system, the throughput of the system for the same key size increases linearly with the number of keys whereas the condition in a CPU+GPU system is one where the throughput is much better. But in the case of a GPU only initially throughput is humongous when compared to the former but it degrades when the number of keys is increased. This is due to the limitations of the GPU memory which is for a large number of keys CPU+GPU is preferred. GPU+CPU methods throughput also decreases when the number of keys is drastically increased but it is still 5 times higher than that of CPU.

For a scalable Blockchain-based EHR storage and query system, we can use the CPU+GPU combination if the radix tree is considered to be implemented, here as informed before the search complexity is the binary search of the key size i.e., O(k) k is the key size. Whereas if you choose a hash-based lookup table the complexity is O (1) but the system must be designed such that collision and its effects are minimized. If those precautions are not included the performance will decrease exponentially.

CONCLUSION

In this chapter, a proposal has been made to accelerate Blockchain-based EHR search and retrieval in the form of key-value pairs and has also explored how GPUs could be used to bring about more efficient implementations of the same system. A Radix Tree based structure and a Hash Table based structure have both been implemented and compared to the base case of a Linked List structure and the improvements in insertion into KVS and the search performance have been represented graphically we have a clear upward trend in the same.

The current scope of this chapter is parallel and efficient read access to the Blockchain-based EHR data that is being collected. The proposed structure facilitates a much more efficient read access time for the data than the already existing methods. The structure used can be modified based on the size, availability, and replication factors as demanded by the users so that the best performance can be achieved.

REFERENCES

[1] Nakamoto, Satoshi. (2006). Bitcoin. *"A Peer-to-Peer Electronic Cash System."* Bitcoin.org. https://bitcoin.org/bitcoin.pdf.

[2] Hetherington, Tayler, and Rogers, Timothy and Hsu, Lisa and O'Connor, Mike & Aamodt, Tor. (2012). *"Characterizing and evaluating a key-value store application on heterogeneous CPU-GPU systems."* ISPASS 2012 - IEEE International Symposium on

Performance Analysis of Systems and Software. doi: 10.1109/ ISPASS.2012.6189209.

[3] Karras, Tero. (2012). "Maximizing Parallelism in the Construction of BVHs, Octrees, and k-d Trees." *Proceedings of the Fourth ACM SIGGRAPH/Eurographics conference on High-Performance Graphics*, 33-37. doi: 10.2312/EGGH/HPG12/033-037.

[4] Leis, V., Kemper, Alfons. & Neumann, Thomas. (2013). "The adaptive radix tree: ARTful indexing for main-memory databases". *Proceedings - International Conference on Data Engineering*, 38-49. doi: 10.1109/ICDE.2013.6544812.

[5] Gavin Wood. (2014). "*Ethereum: A Secure Decentralized Generalised Transaction Ledger.*" North American Bitcoin Conference (Jan 2014). https://gavwood.com/paper.pdf.

[6] Liu, Dapengand Cui, Zengdiand Xu, Shaochunand Liu, Huafu. (2014). *"An empirical study on the performance of hash table."* 2014 IEEE/ACIS 13th International Conference on Computer and Information Science, ICIS 2014 – Proceedings: 477-484. doi: 10. 1109/ICIS.2014.6912180.

[7] Morishima, Shin. & Matsutani, Hiroki. (2014). *"Performance Evaluations of Graph Database using CUDA and OpenMP Compatible Libraries."* ACM SIGARCH Computer Architecture News. 42. 75-80. doi: 10.1145/2693714.2693728.

[8] Hetherington, Tayler, O'Connor, Mike. & Aamodt, Tor. (2015). *"MemcachedGPU: Scaling-up Scale-out Key-value Stores."* SoCC '15: Proceedings of the Sixth ACM Symposium on Cloud Computing (August 2015): 43–57 doi: 10.1145/2806777.2806836.

[9] Azaria, Asaph. Ekblaw, Ariel, Vieira, Thiago, & Lippman, Andrew. (2016). *"MedRec: Using Blockchain for Medical Data Access and Permission Management,"* 2nd International Conference on Open and Big Data (OBD) (Vienna, 2016): 25-30. doi: 10.1109/OBD. 2016.11.

[10] Morishima, Shin & Matsutani, Hiroki. (2018). *"Accelerating Blockchain Search of Full Nodes Using GPUs,"* 26th Euromicro International Conference on Parallel, Distributed and Network-based

Processing (PDP), Cambridge, 2018: 244-248, doi: 10.1109/PDP2018.2018.00041.

[11] Pungila, Ciprian & Negru, Viorel. (2020). *"Improving Blockchain Security Validation and Transaction Processing Through Heterogeneous Computing."* International Joint Conference: 12th International Conference on Computational Intelligence in Security for Information Systems (CISIS 2019) and 10th International Conference on European Transnational Education (ICEUTE 2019). CISIS 2019, ICEUTE 2019. *Advances in Intelligent Systems and Computing*, vol 951. Springer, Cham doi: 10.1007/978-3-030-20005-3_14.

[12] Lemieux, Victoria, Hofman, Darra, Batista, Danielle & Joo, Alysha. (2019). *"Blockchain Technology and Recordkeeping."* Arma international Educational Foundation (May 2019) http://armaedfoundation.org/wp-content/uploads/2019/06/AIEF-Research-Paper-Blockchain-Technology-Recordkeeping.pdf.

[13] Mahony, Aidan & Popovici, Emanuel. (2019). *"A Systematic Review of Blockchain Hardware Acceleration Architectures,"* 30th Irish Signals and Systems Conference (ISSC), Maynooth, Ireland, 2019: 1-6. doi: 10.1109/ISSC.2019.8904936.

[14] Shahnaz, Ayesha, Qamar, Usman & Khalid, Ayesha. (2019). *"Using Blockchain for Electronic Health Records," IEEE Access*, vol. 7, (2019), 147782-147795. doi: 10.1109/ACCESS.2019.2946373.

[15] Nvidia Corporation. (2007). *"CUDA C++ Programming Guide."* https://docs.nvidia.com/pdf/CUDA_C_Programming_Guide.pdf.

[16] LevelDB. (2011). *"LevelDB."* https://dbdb.io/db/leveldb.

[17] California Health and Human Services. (2019). *"Electronic Health Record (EHR) Incentive Program Payments."* https://data.world/chhs/579fbb1f-0078-4fe3-9bc8-c09d91ad3589.

In: Computing Paradigms for Smart Healthcare ISBN: 978-1-53618-619-2
Editors: B. Vinoth Kumar et al.

Chapter 10

SECURE CRYPTOGRAPHIC KEY EXCHANGE BETWEEN BODY AREA SENSORS

R. Rekha*[*]*, PhD

Department of Information Technology, PSG College of Technology, Coimbatore

ABSTRACT

A Wireless Body Area Sensor Network (WBASN) is a network of small wearable sensing devices that helps to monitor the health condition of patients in a continuous manner. It is necessary for the sensing devices to collect the sensed information and forward it to a hub, which is another wearable device on the body of the patient to perform processing of collected data. The medical data should not be transmitted in clear form and must be encrypted using cryptographic key. This chapter discusses a Fast Fourier Transform, prediction filter and linear coding-based method to agree upon the cryptographic key required to encrypt /decrypt the collected medical data among sensors of same patient body during transmission. Experimental results show that using the proposed method

[*] Corresponding Author Email: rekha.psgtech@gmail.com.

the Half Total Error Rate was achieved to be 0.21. This can be further improved by choice of suitable error control coding techniques in future.

Keywords: body area sensor network, cryptographic key, key agreement, fast fourier transform, prediction filter, error control coding

INTRODUCTION

Cardio Vascular Disease (CVD) has become the important cause of death all over the world. CVD is chronic in nature since it lasts for longer duration and it needs continuous monitoring her by healthcare professionals. Some of the other examples of chronic diseases include diabetes, asthma and cancer. Insisting patients with chronic diseases in hospital will lead to increase in healthcare cost and other practical limitations. Remote Patient Monitoring (RPM) systems helps patients with chronic diseases to be remotely monitored with the help of small biosensors which are worn or implanted on the body of the patient. Medical data collected with the help of such biosensors, send the collected information to a central hub where the data gets processed. This way of exchanging information between sensors placed on same patient's body is referred as intra-sensor communication. The processed information will reach the healthcare professionals for further decision.

The main problem faced by the remote patient monitoring system is to preserve the privacy of the health-related information. There are chances for the medical information to be received by intruders when sent in clear form. Hence the information needs to be encrypted and then transmitted to the receiver. Symmetric cryptosystems require a cryptographic key to be shared among the sender and receiver units. To achieve secure intra-sensor communication, both the sender and receiver should share a common cryptographic key. The principal issue faced by BASN is in adding a cryptographic key generator in the smaller size, low power, and low computational ability biosensors. Hence there is a need for finding alternate mechanism for key generation and agreement between communication sensors.

This chapter begins with a brief introduction to remote patient monitoring system and the challenges faced by it during intra-sensor communication. Introduction is followed by a detailed survey on methods discussed by researchers to establish secure intra-sensor communication. A new method based on Fast Fourier Transform (FFT), Linear prediction and error control coding was explained in the next section followed by implementation results and analysis.

LITERATURE SURVEY

Several researchers have discussed biometric based key generation and key agreement between communicating sensors in BASN. Electrocardiogram (ECG) signals were used for key generation and for key distribution among communicating sensors by [1]. The authors also proved that ECG signals provide key with good randomness. A fuzzy scheme along with ECG based features was used by [2] for key agreement between sending and receiving sensors. Since both the sensors are located on the same patient body, the features generated by both the sensors will be almost similar. But in order to agree upon a common key, the slight mismatch should be rectified. Hence the authors propose a fuzzy scheme which compensates for the slight variation in agreed features. Additional random points were added along with the original features to avoid the intruders to guess the genuine points. The drawback of this method is the memory required while adding random points to valid points. This is avoided by "Improved Jules Sudan" proposed by [3]. Instead of additional random points, the authors proposed to use a tolerance parameter to compensate for feature mismatch. A similar approach in which a coffer was generated along with the existing approach of transmitting valid features generated with ECG signal and chaff points was proposed by [4]. The drawback of this system is the memory overhead. Several research works by [5, 6] made use of ECG signal for secure key agreement. Prediction techniques were used for key agreement by [7, 8]. Literature survey on systems that use biometrics for key generation and key agreement is tabulated in Table 1.

Table 1. Literature survey on biometrics for key generation and key agreement

Literature	Implication
[9]	The authors experimented with capturing several biometric features from distinct locations of the human body. Cryptographic keys were generated using fusion of several biometric traits and concluded that the biometric based key generation have enough randomness to be used a s cryptographic key.
[10]	The authors experimented with key generation using the ECG signal captured at distinct locations of same person. The results show that the Inter Pulse Interval in ECG signal can be used for key generation. They also concluded that keys generated at distinct locations vary slightly.
[1]	Multi point fuzzy scheme was used by the authors for key agreement. The experimental results also show that ECG signals can provide key with sufficient randomness to be used as cryptographic key.
[11]	The authors generated key using entity identifiers which are further produced with the help of IPI of ECG signals. The limitation of this approach is its slight increase in computational complexity.
[12]	The authors experimented with fusion of both static biometric such as finger print and dynamic biometric trait such as ECG signal. It was concluded in their research work that unique cryptographic keys can be generated using this approach.

Literature	Implication
[13]	The authors experimented with key generation using both ECG signal and the derivative of the ECG signal. They were able to prove that the keys are unique and the number of bits that differ between keys generated using ECG signals of different persons was more than 50 bits.
[2]	Fuzzy based scheme was used to agree upon a common key between communicating sensors. The drawback of this system was that the system is vulnerable to correlation attack. Hence genuine points transmitted from sender can be guessed by intruder by correlating two vaults from sender.
[14]	The authors were able to agree upon common key by sharing secret among communicating implanted medical sensors before intra-sensor communication. The drawback was its time complexity.
[3]	The authors introduced a concept of tolerance parameter for symmetric key agreement. The advantage of this method is that it does not require any secret to be shared before key agreement and additional points are not needed.
[4]	Over lapping segments of ECG signals were used by authors for key generation. This method does not require any prior secret sharing between communicating sensors.

METHODOLOGY

The objective of the research work is to securely agree upon a common key between the various body area sensors on a patient body. Assumption is made that all the sensors connected on patient body are also able to capture ECG signal along with its ability to capture its desired physiological signal. If sensor A wants to communicate with sensor B, then it must first share a symmetric key with sensor B for possible encryption and transmission of physiological data. The concept of Differential Pulse Code Modulation is used in this work for key sharing. The block diagram of the method is shown in figure 1.

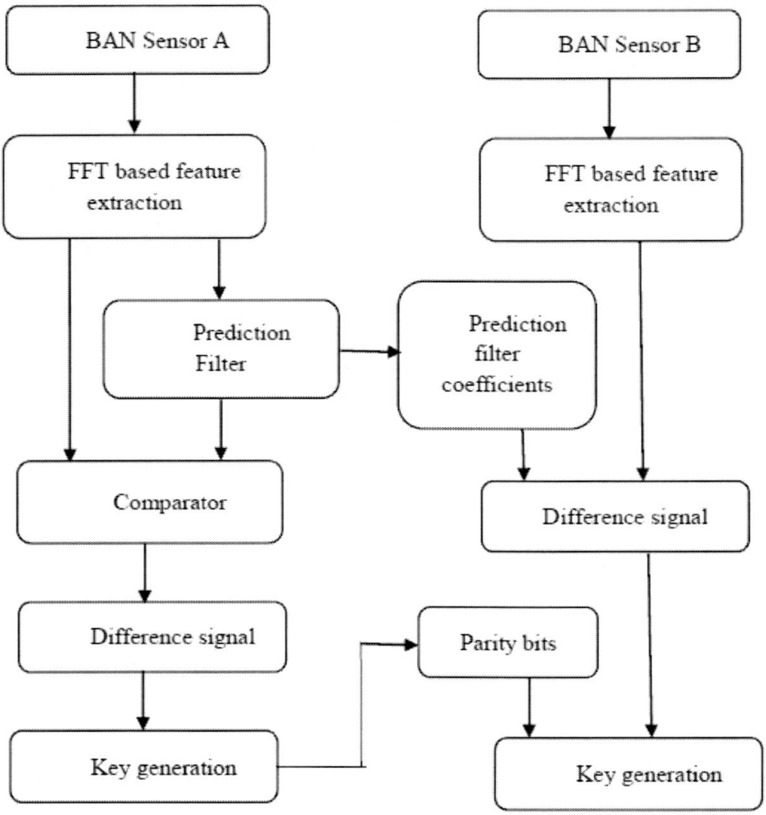

Figure 1. Block diagram of secure key agreement technique.

The principle followed to achieve this task is as follows:Firstly, the sender node and receiver node starts capturing the ECG signal for few seconds simultaneously. Features are extracted by both sender and receiver node from the captured ECG signal using Fast Fourier Transform (FFT). Sender node then tries to find the predicted version of original FFT signal with the help of Prediction filter. The difference between the original signal and predicted signal is computed and quantized to get the output in the form of a binary code. This binary code will be used as the symmetric key. The receiver will also try to compute the error signal between its own version of original signal at receiver side and predicted signal obtained with the help of prediction coefficients shared from sender. Few differences between the binary codes generated between sender and receiver are rectified with the help of linear block coding technique.

a) Feature Extraction

Sender and receiver nodes of WBASN collect ECG signals simultaneously for a duration of ten seconds. Collected ECG signals are sampled at a sampling rate of 60 Hz. Fast Fourier Transform (FFT) is performed over the samples. Fourier Transform decomposes a signal into complex exponential functions and expresses it in terms of different frequencies of the waves that make up the signal. Any deviations in the regular shape of the normal ECG beat can be easily visualized by analyzing the frequency content of the ECG segment. This work uses Fast Fourier transform (FFT) for feature extraction.

b) Differential Quantization

The adjacent samples of the FFT signal may show redundancy. Hence, by knowing the past behavior of samples, the current sample can be predicted with the help of prediction filter. The prediction filter coefficients are selected in such a way that the Mean Square Error (MSE) between the actual signal and predicted signal is minimum. This difference between the actual and predicted sample is quantized and converted to binary sequence which can be used as the key for cryptographic process.

Let x[n] be the actual sample and $\widehat{x[n]}$ be the predicted sample, then the quantization error is given by, q[n] = x[n] - $\widehat{x[n]}$. The predicted output by the prediction filter is obtained as,$\widehat{x[n]} = \sum_{k=1}^{p} w_k x[n-k]$, where ‘p’ is the order of prediction filter, w_k is the filter coefficients and x[n-k] is the delayed version of actual input samples.

c) Key Generation

The difference signal is quantized and the output obtained is converted to binary sequence. If the quantized value is greater than '0', then the bit generated in key is '1' and if the quantized value is lesser than or equal to '0', then the bit generated in key is '1'. By this process, a 128 bit key is generated at the sender. This key is divided into small blocks of size 'k' and parity bits of size 'n-k' are added with each block to construct code words of size 'n'. The 'n-k' parity bits and the prediction filter coefficients are sent to the receiver for common key agreement.

d) Key Agreement

The receiver receives the prediction filter coefficients and parity bits from the sender. It generates its own features from the ECG signal captured at receiver side. The key generation at receiver side is performed by generating the difference signal with the help of its own FFT signal and predicted signal with the help of prediction filter coefficients received. The obtained binary key may have few mismatching bits with respect to the key generated at sender side. This difference is corrected with the help of parity bits received from the sender.

Experimental Results

The dataset used for experimentation was taken from Physionet/MIT_BIH Arrhythmia database. The MIT-BIH Arrhythmia Database contains 48 half-hour excerpts of two-channel ambulatory ECG recordings, obtained from 47 subjects studied by the BIH Arrhythmia Laboratory between 1975 and 1979. MATLAB R2020a is used for experimental trials. A sample ECG signal recorded for ten seconds from patient id: 100 is shown in figure 2.

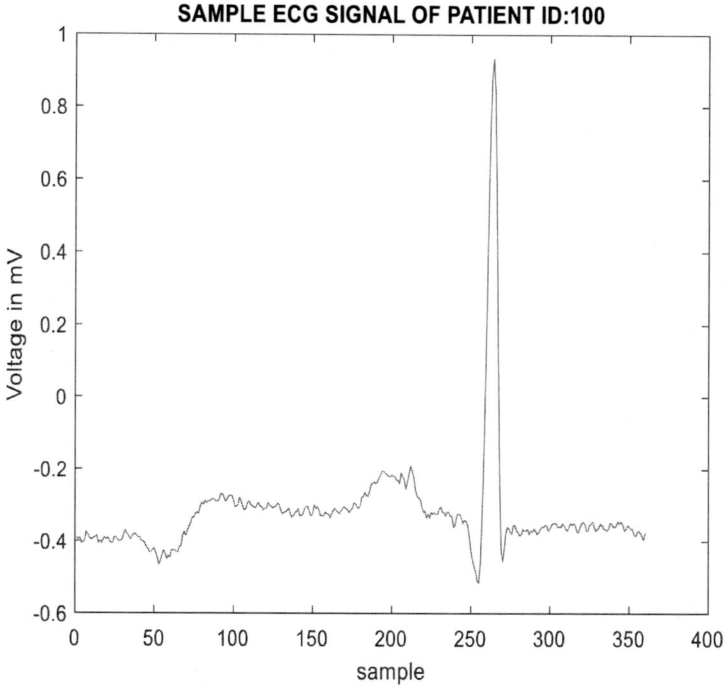

Figure 2. Sample ECG signal.

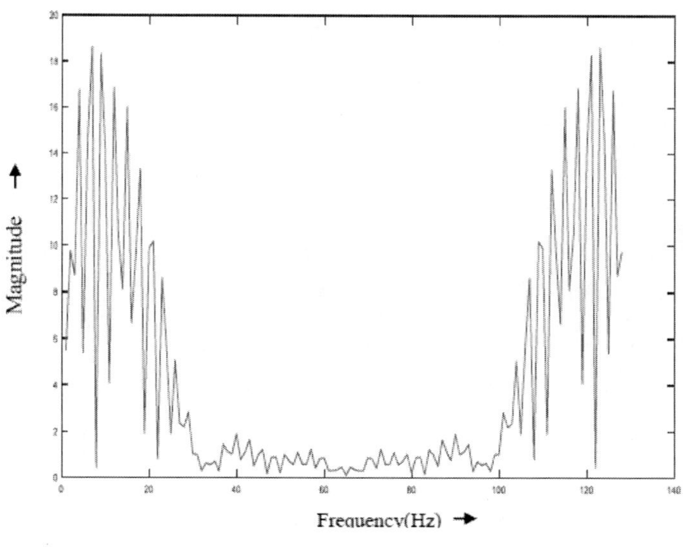

Figure 3. FFT of captured ECG signal.

The features are extracted from captured ECG signal using Fast Fourier Transform and the FFT output is shown in figure 3.

Selection of appropriate prediction filter order is particularly important in achieving the objective of minimum mean square error between the actual and predicted signal. After experimentation, it was found that filter order of '3' gives better result. The plot of actual signal and predicted version of original signal using prediction filter of order '3' is shown in figure 4. On an average the hamming distance between the keys generated by sender and receiver of same Body Area Network is 11, while the hamming distance between the keys generated by sensors of different Body Area Networks is 49. Hence, to achieve symmetric key between sender and receiver, linear error control coding technique is used. Larger the number of parity bits that are added with block of binary sequence, greater its error correcting capability. At the same time, addition of more parity bits may also lead to increase the false acceptance rate. Adding lesser number of parity bits with the binary sequence block may lead to increase in false rejection rate. Hence optimum number of redundant/parity bits should be added to the binary blocks to reduce both false acceptance and rejection rates.

EVALUATION METRICS

The metrics used to evaluate the research work are defined as follows:

- False Acceptance Rate (FAR) is a measure of the likelihood that the system will falsely accept an access by an unauthorized user.
- False Rejection Rate (FRR) is a measure of the likelihood that the system will falsely reject an access by an authorized user.

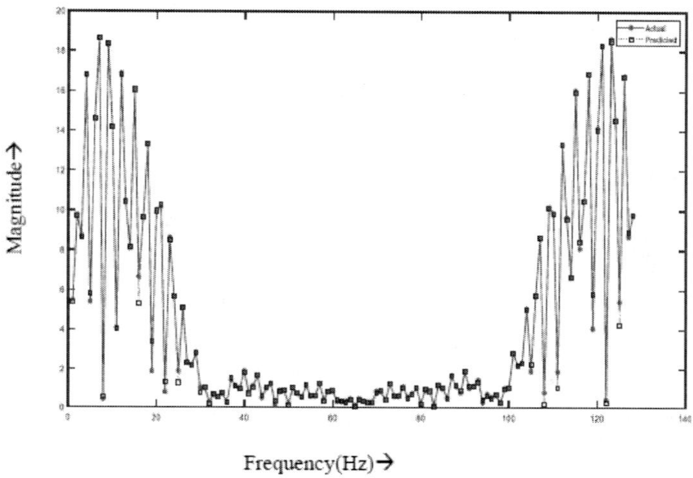

Figure 4. Actual and predicted signal at sender node.

The experimental results show that addition of more number of redundant bits lead to increase in false acceptance rate. Lesser number of parity bits led to increase in false rejection rate. The optimum number of redundant bits helps to get a FAR and FRR of 0.21. This is shown in figure 5.

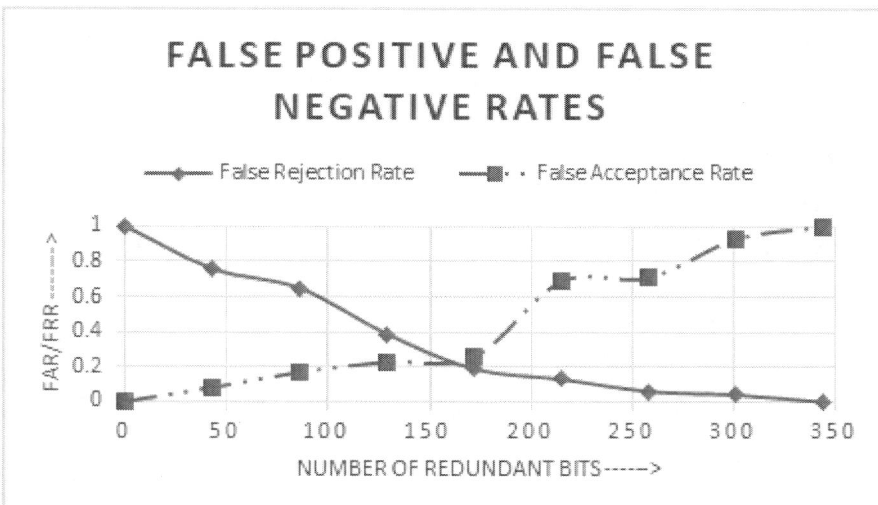

Figure 5. False positive and false negative rates.

Advantages of proposed method:

- The proposed system transmits only the prediction filter coefficients and redundant / parity bits to the receiver. Hence it is not possible for an intruder to find the symmetric key without knowing the ECG signal to make prediction.
- The proposed system do not need any vault to hide the secret key while transmission from sender to receiver.
- Possibility of replay attack is not possible since ECG signal captured at a time instant will not be the same after some time duration.
- The proposed method do not involve with any complex procedures such as polynomial construction or reconstruction. Hence computational overhead is reduced.

CONCLUSION

Differential pulse code modulation and linear block coding based symmetric key agreement scheme has been proposed and experimented. The experimental results shows that the hamming distance between the keys generated at sensor nodes of same Body Area Network is very less. Hence it can be corrected using any of the error control coding techniques such as Linear Block Codes, BCH or Reed Solomon Codes. The proposed method greatly reduces the computational overhead compared to other fuzzy vault techniques and eliminates replay attacks during wireless transmission of medical data.

REFERENCES

[1] Bui, Francis Minhthang, and Dimitrios Hatzinakos. "Biometric methods for secure communications in body sensor networks:

resource-efficient key management and signal-level data scrambling." *EURASIP Journal on Advances in Signal Processing* 2008 (2007): 1-16.

[2] Venkatasubramanian, Krishna K., Ayan Banerjee, and Sandeep Kumar S. Gupta. "PSKA: Usable and secure key agreement scheme for body area networks." *IEEE Transactions on Information Technology in Biomedicine* 14, no. 1 (2009): 60-68.

[3] Zhang, Zhaoyang, Honggang Wang, Athanasios V. Vasilakos, and Hua Fang. "ECG-cryptography and authentication in body area networks." *IEEE Transactions on Information Technology in Biomedicine* 16, no. 6 (2012): 1070-1078.

[4] Hu, Chunqiang, Xiuzhen Cheng, Fan Zhang, Dengyuan Wu, Xiaofeng Liao, and Dechang Chen. "OPFKA: Secure and efficient ordered-physiological-feature-based key agreement for wireless body area networks." In *2013 Proceedings IEEE INFOCOM*, pp. 2274-2282. IEEE, 2013.

[5] Tang, Wenjuan, Kuan Zhang, Ju Ren, Yaoxue Zhang, and Xuemin Shen. "Flexible and efficient authenticated key agreement scheme for BANs based on physiological features." *IEEE Transactions on Mobile Computing* 18, no. 4 (2018): 845-856.

[6] Tang, Wenjuan, Kuan Zhang, Deyu Zhang, Ju Ren, Yaoxue Zhang, and Xuemin Sherman Shen. "Fog-enabled smart health: Toward cooperative and secure healthcare service provision." *IEEE Communications Magazine* 57, no. 5 (2019): 42-48.

[7] Zaghouani, Emna Kalai, Abderrazak Jemai, Adel Benzina, and Rabah Attia. "ELPA: A new key agreement scheme based on linear prediction of ECG features for WBAN." In *2015 23rd European Signal Processing Conference (EUSIPCO)*, pp. 81-85. IEEE, 2015.

[8] Zaghouani, Emna Kalai, Adel Benzina, and Rabah Attia. "ECG based authentication for e-healthcare systems: Towards a secured ECG features transmission." In *2017 13th International Wireless Communications and Mobile Computing Conference (IWCMC)*, pp. 1777-1783. IEEE, 2017.

[9] Cherukuri, Sriram, Krishna K. Venkatasubramanian, and Sandeep KS Gupta. "Biosec: A biometric based approach for securing communication in wireless networks of biosensors implanted in the human body." In *2003 International Conference on Parallel Processing Workshops, 2003. Proceedings.*, pp. 432-439. IEEE, 2003.

[10] Poon, Carmen CY, Yuan-Ting Zhang, and Shu-Di Bao. "A novel biometrics method to secure wireless body area sensor networks for telemedicine and m-health." *IEEE Communications Magazine* 44, no. 4 (2006): 73-81.

[11] Bao, Shu-Di, Carmen CY Poon, Yuan-Ting Zhang, and Lian-Feng Shen. "Using the timing information of heartbeats as an entity identifier to secure body sensor network." *IEEE transactions on information technology in biomedicine* 12, no. 6 (2008): 772-779.

[12] Zhang, G. H., Carmen CY Poon, and Y. T. Zhang. "A biometrics-based security solution for encryption and authentication in tele-healthcare systems." In *2009 2nd International Symposium on Applied Sciences in Biomedical and Communication Technologies*, pp. 1-4. IEEE, 2009.

[13] Zhang, G. H., Carmen CY Poon, and Y. T. Zhang. "A fast key generation method based on dynamic biometrics to secure wireless body sensor networks for p-health." In *2010 Annual International Conference of the IEEE Engineering in Medicine and Biology*, pp. 2034-2036. IEEE, 2010.

[14] Xu, Fengyuan, Zhengrui Qin, Chiu C. Tan, Baosheng Wang, and Qun Li. "IMDGuard: Securing implantable medical devices with the external wearable guardian." In *2011 Proceedings IEEE INFOCOM*, pp. 1862-1870. IEEE, 2011.

About the Editors

Dr B Vinoth Kumar
Associate Professor
Department of Information Technology, PSG College of Technology,
Coimbatore, Tamil Nadu, India

Dr. B.Vinoth Kumar is working as an Associate Professor with 16 years of experience in the Department of Information Technology at PSG College of Technology. His research interests include Soft Computing, Blockchain and Digital Image Processing. He is a Life Member of the Institution of Engineers- India (IEI), International Association of Engineers (IAENG) and Indian Society of Systems for Science and Engineering (ISSE). He is author of more than 26 papers in refereed journals and international conferences. He has edited three books with reputed publishers such as Springer and CRC Press. He serves as a Guest Editor/Reviewer of many journals with leading publishers such as Inderscience, De Gruyter and Springer. He has received a research grant of 40 Lakhs from Department of Science and Technology (DST)-India.

Dr J Uma Maheswari
Assistant Professor
Department of Computer Science and Engineering,
PSG College of Technology, Coimbatore, Tamil Nadu, India

Dr. J Uma Maheswari is an Assistant Professor(SG) with 13 years of experience in Computer Science and Engineering in PSG College of Technology. She completed her BE Computer Science and Engineering in Sri Krishna College of Engineering and Technology, Coimbatore from Bharathiar University in 2003 and ME Computer Science and Engineering in JJ College of Engineering and Technology, Trichy from Anna University in 2006. Her areas of research include Computing and Semantic web services. She has received a research grant of 43 lakhs from esteemed agencies like AICTE and DST. She has edited a book with reputed publisher such CRC Press.

Dr G R Karpagam
Professor and Associate Head
Department of Computer Science and Engineering,
PSG College of Technology, Coimbatore, Tamil Nadu, India

Dr. G R Karpagam is a Professor and Associate Head with 24 years of experience in Computer Science and Engineering in PSG College of Technology. She obtained her BE, ME, and PhD in Computer Science and Engineering. She also heads PSG-GRD Memorial Library and has guided 6 PhDs in the area of SOA and web services. She is a Senior IEEE member and is operating as the Vice Chair of ACM, local Chapter. She is a recipient of the PSG & Sons Teacher of the Year Award. She has set up several state-of- Art laboratories funded by Industries and Funding agencies. They include Center for Artificial Intelligence Research (AIR), SOA and Cloud Computing, Open source. She has received a research grant to a tune of 3 Crores from esteemed agencies such as DST, DBT, AICTE and UGC, Cognizant, Cordys, Impiger and Hewlett Packard Enterprise Her areas of specialization are DBMS, Data Structures and

Algorithms, Web services, Cloud Computing, Machine learning and Blockchain. She serves as a reviewer and editor for peer reviewed National and International conferences and journals. She has published 100+ papers in journals and conferences and is editor of two books with publishers being Springer and CRC press.

Dr P Sivakumar
Assistant Professor
Department of Electrical and Electronics Engineering,
PSG College of Technology, Coimbatore, Tamil Nadu, India

Dr. P Sivakumar is working as a Selection grade Assistant Professor with 10 years of experience in the Department of Electrical and Electronics Engineering at PSG College of Technology. His research interests include Model Based Design of Automotive Software, Computational Intelligence and Image Processing. He is a Life Member of the Institution of Engineers-India (IEI) and International Association of Engineers (IAENG). He is author of more than 15 papers in refereed journals and international conferences. He has reviewed the 8th edition of a book titled "Understanding of Automotive Electronics" Elsevier. He serves as a Guest Editor/Reviewer of many journals with leading publishers such as Inderscience and Springer.

INDEX

D

E

F

G

H

I

J

K

L

M

N

T

U

V

W

X

Z